AF394724

STYLED

Sally Mackinnon is one of Australia's most beloved and experienced personal stylists, having launched her business Styled by Sally in Melbourne in 2007. With her natural eye for style and down to earth, intuitive and personable approach, Sally has helped thousands of clients look and feel their best.

As well as providing one-to-one personal shopping, styling and wardrobe consultations, Sally delivers inclusive styling content around seasonal updates, new interpretations of timeless trends, and rules that were made to be broken to her 250K-plus followers on Instagram @styledbysally. Above all else, Sally passionately believes we should wear what makes us feel good, offering practical and realistic advice to suit every budget and lifestyle.

Sally is a regular consultant to mainstream media appearing across major television networks, a favoured brand ambassador for local and international retailers, and a featured panellist at fashion events across the country.

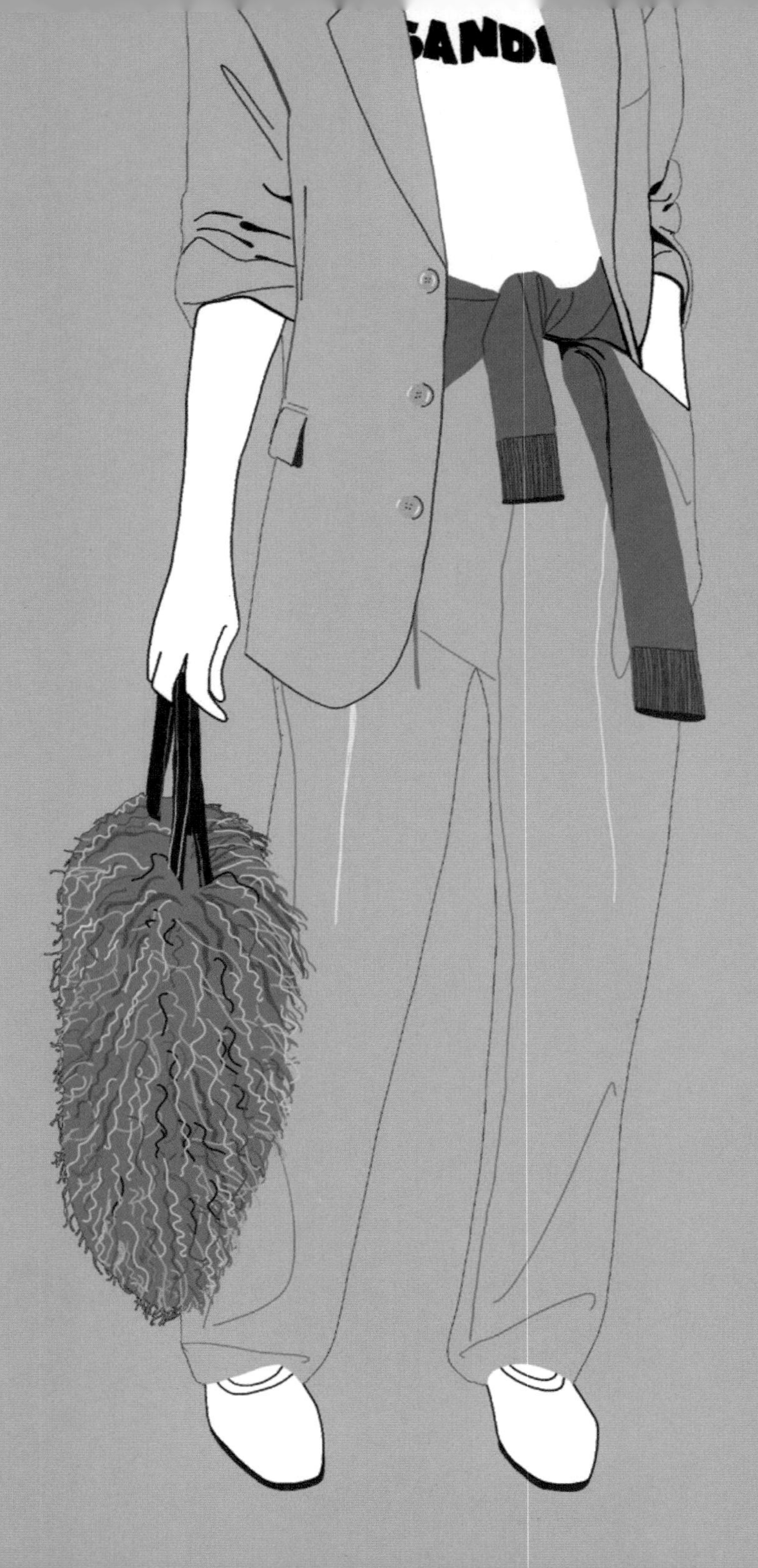

SANDI

STYLED

How to dress as your most stylish self

Sally Mackinnon

Illustrations by Juliet Sulejmani

Thank you to my 30-something self who trusted her gut, believed in herself and followed her passion, and who brought me to all the women I've met since. If I hadn't got to know each of you, listen to you and style you, there would be no book. You are my endless inspiration. Always, and in style.

CONTENTS

Every woman has
the power to create
a style that reflects
her *personality*,
her *passions*
and her *purpose*.

INTRODUCTION

Hello and welcome to *STYLED*. I'm so thrilled you're here so we can delve deeper into the insider secrets I share with you on social media, learnt over my twenty years as a personal stylist. I work with real women every day to help them gain confidence in expressing themselves through what they wear. It might sound like a stretch but I have been told countless times that finding their style has helped my clients live bigger, better, happier lives. And when you really think about it, it makes sense. In a world where trends come and go, personal style remains a timeless expression of who you are. Finding your style involves a process of determining what you love about yourself and how to highlight that. It's not about fitting into a mould or following the latest trends – it's about embracing your individuality and showcasing your inner, true self. Every woman has the power to create a style that reflects her personality, her passions and her purpose. This book is your guide to discovering and celebrating that, empowering you to step out with confidence and into the joy of being unapologetically you.

Styled by Sally

Before I set up my business, Styled by Sally, I was a schoolteacher and to this day I still get asked, 'How did you make the transition from schoolteacher to personal stylist?' The answer is quite straightforward.

As a teacher I imparted knowledge, encouraged my students to explore ideas, helped them learn new skills and information, supported them when they made mistakes, nurtured them to try new things and praised them when they did their best. I loved this but after I had been teaching for around thirteen years, I needed a change. Taking my long service leave, I decided to travel solo for six months, starting out in the European summer and ending in the American winter. In October, I landed in New York City for the very first time, and it was love at first sight. The weather was starting to cool and typically the days were a mild 20-odd degrees Celsius, perfect for walking the streets of Manhattan, which I did a lot of.

It was peak *Sex in the City* era so, naturally, I'd booked a tour, which started somewhere near Central Park. To get there I walked along Fifth Avenue from Downtown. I still remember all the different neighbourhoods I walked through, and their distinctive vibes, each unique, from one block to the next.

Given the show's emphasis on fashion, and my love of it, I dressed carefully from my limited wardrobe. After nearly four months of travelling out of a backpack I'd become inventive with layering, and throughout my journey had changed my pack's contents to match the weather. As it had turned colder, I'd tossed out a few worn-out summer staples and replaced them with brown knee-high boots, tights and a warm, belted jacket.

Though I'd come from working in a profession that was a far cry from fashion, getting dressed, putting outfits together and knowing what worked (and what didn't) had always come naturally to me. My friends often asked me to accompany them on shopping trips to help them buy a pair of jeans, find an outfit for an occasion or simply choose what to wear for a night out.

I will never forget a parent–teacher interview with a Year 5 boy's mother. Jarvis was a great kid, shy and quiet but always engaged and eager to please. The first thing his mum said, before I had a chance to tell her what a great student her son was, was that every night he would describe what shoes I had worn, in great detail! Let's just say my love of a good shoe was within me well before I even knew I would one day become a fashion stylist.

On that day, back on the *Sex and the City* tour, my boots became the core of my outfit. Styled with the black 'walking shorts' I'd worn throughout summer, the boots and tights were the perfect replacement for strappy sandals. Up top, I wore a few layers, finishing off the look with my new brown-tweed belted jacket. I was warm and comfortable and felt stylish (as much as one can, dressing out of a backpack!).

The tour host asked us all to introduce ourselves and say where we were from.

'My name is Sally and I'm from Melbourne, Australia,' I said when it was my turn.

'Oh,' she said, surprised. 'I saw you earlier today walking down Fifth Avenue and thought to myself, look at that stylish New Yorker!'

To say I was surprised and flattered is an understatement! But that was the moment I realised my life was about to change. When I arrived at my next destination, Canada, I emailed my school principal and asked to work a four-day week when I got home. I knew I needed to give styling a real go. Exactly twelve months after that day, I officially launched Styled by Sally and booked my first client. And just over twelve months later, at the end of 2008, I left teaching to pursue a full-time career as a personal stylist.

The adjustment was not as dramatic as it sounds. As a personal stylist I also teach, listen, adapt, support and educate. I use the same skills and approach I needed for teaching, just applied to a different topic! The lovely difference is that I get to teach people from all walks of life – from teenagers to retirees,

CEOs to stay-at-home mums, politicians to police. Regardless of someone's job, status or budget, they all come to me with the same common goal: to feel good in their clothes.

Was I born with a natural eye for style? I think so. I'd always been interested in clothes and fashion, from styling my Barbie dolls to setting up fashion shoots with my sister in the family lounge room!

But that doesn't mean I've always been confident in my personal style. Like many of us, I stumbled my way through my teenage years, not really having the self-confidence to express myself through my clothing. Being a tall, shy young woman, I hated feeling 'obvious', so I'd cover myself up by wearing oversized clothing (which, luckily for me, was also 'on trend' at the time). The lessons I learnt from styling myself, I now use to help others develop theirs. I have tried all the tricks, learnt all the rules (then tossed away most), and honed my natural instinct with decades of constant learning to distill all this down into useful, practical tips for you.

What to expect from *STYLED*

I want *STYLED* to be a source of inspiration for anyone coming to it at any point in time – whether that's today as you're reading this, or twenty years from now when it's been handed down to a daughter or picked up in a second-hand bookshop. While your style will change over time, my tips and philosophies are steadfast and can be applied throughout your life as your personal style evolves. It's advice that I hope will resonate, whatever your size, shape, height, age or budget. If you can take one thing from this book and apply it in a way that makes your life easier, ensures your wardrobe works harder, and helps you hold your head higher, then this is going to be worth the read. Whatever your job, wherever you live or wherever in life you happen to be, *STYLED* has been written for you.

Throughout the book, I'll give you little tasks to complete and questions to answer. The aim of these practical activities is to help you define your style, identify your personal needs, prioritise your wardrobe purpose and shop with intention. There are *no* wrong answers, just ideas, exploration, solutions and outcomes.

We'll look at outfit building, wardrobe organising and inspiration sourcing. I'll share my insider tips on how to shop like a pro and the style hacks I've learnt over the years that will be game changers for your life. You'll learn why age is irrelevant when it comes to personal style, how to listen to your feelings and not anyone else's, and how to get dressed without rules.

I'll share the experiences of real-life clients (with names changed to protect their privacy) that you'll be able to relate to. The illustrations by

Juliet Sulejmani (@thejulietreport) are a crucial part of the book too.
I decided upon using illustrations instead of photographs of real people for
a couple of reasons. First, I loved collaborating with Juliet on my signature
graphic tee and wanted to work with her again! And second, because an
illustration holds no preconceived beliefs or association with any one
person. As such, you'll note that each figure has a nondescript complexion
and facial features – a blank canvas if you will – upon which to project
your own experience. When you look at these illustrations I want you to see
yourselves, not an actor, model or celebrity who happens to be notable today
but your own true, spectacular self. If there's one takeout message I want
to give you with this book, it's to unapologetically express, celebrate and
appreciate you! And everything I share here with you has been created with
the intention of helping you do that.

My hope for this book is that it will guide and inspire you to dress in any way
you want, giving you the tools and permission to do so. It's an extension of
the everyday conversations I've had with my clients for many years. I want
to teach you how to trust your own feelings and instincts when it comes to
your personal style. Don't feel good in a colour? Don't wear it! Don't like that
trend? Ignore it! When you leave the house, what outfits make you feel most
'you'? When you go to work, which outfits leave you feeling capable, seen,
heard? When you catch up with friends, which outfit consistently invites
compliments? The practical tips I share have the potential to change the
way you think and feel about your clothes, because 'What am I going to wear
today?' is a question we all ask ourselves. You will learn how to listen to this
intuition to help you formulate a personal style that feels right. One outfit at
a time. Every day.

I want to teach
   you how to trust
your own *feelings*
and *instincts* when
it comes to your
   personal style.

One

Foundations of Style

To put it simply:
clothing is *functional*,
fashion is *fun*
and style is how we
combine the two
to *creatively express
our identity*.

1. DEVELOP YOUR STYLE AND PURPOSE

Personal style is . . . what exactly?

Style is such a broad term. As we work through this book, we'll build up layers of knowledge and insights around it. There's so much I can (and will!) say about style but let's start with this fundamental insight: style is *not* fashion. I love fashion but I don't consider my job as a personal stylist as working 'in' fashion. This book, *STYLED*, is a compendium to my daily job as a personal stylist and here I'll outline what I've learnt through twenty years on the job.

First, you need to develop your style. Fashion is well and good, and we can certainly have fun with it. But well beyond fashion, those people you see who always manage to look good, regardless of where they are or what they are doing, have nailed their personal style.

Personal style is how we express ourselves aesthetically through clothing, accessories, hair and make-up. Personal style is a form of self-expression that allows us to communicate our values and attitudes without saying a word. Our personal style is not static, nor is it set in concrete. Indeed, it can, and arguably should, be fluid – from one day, one occasion, one decade to the next.

Some people seem born with an innate sense of personal style, others may feel like they struggle with it. But whether or not it comes naturally to you, style can most certainly be honed and crafted, as you will learn here. And it's well worth the investment.

Over my career, I've witnessed clothes transform a woman's self-confidence. In the blink of an eye, I've had clients go from actively avoiding the mirror to joyfully giving me permission to post their photo on my social media. I've seen clothing help people land their dream job, attract a life partner and get their midlife mojo back. Our clothing is powerful.

While some may disregard its importance, clothing can fundamentally change the way we feel about ourselves and others. Our clothes and how we wear them are a visual representation of who we are. If we're not there yet, we can use this power to become more like the person we want to be. We can use clothes to help us fit in or make us stand out, to help us feel like we belong or to express our individuality.

But clothing is only part of the equation – I mean, everyone wears clothes, right? But not everyone is stylish. So, how do we become so? Is it simply a matter of keeping up with the latest trends and accessories? Certainly, the retailers would love us to believe that, and of course, I love shopping for new pieces too – it is my job, after all! But knowing what to buy and how to fit it into your existing wardrobe is a skill. Because style is about far more than either clothing or fashion.

To put it simply: clothing is functional, fashion is fun and style is how we combine the two to creatively express our identity. While clothing and fashion work hand in hand and are fundamentally led by brands (though increasingly less so, thanks to social media and market fragmentation), personal style is ultimately up to the individual. Style is the result of the deliberate choices we make when we get dressed. Through these, you can demonstrate your individuality, communicate your personality and view yourself more confidently.

The essence of your style comes down to personal choice. Can you think of anything else in life that allows such generous freedom of expression? What you wear and how you pull it together is totally up to you! Your style choices can be discreet and subtle, or obvious and unmistakable. Even in a uniform, you have some control over how you style it: whether you opt for a looser or tighter fit, and how you button your collar, tuck your top or do your hair.

It's not the individual items you wear that make you stylish but how you piece them together and add accessories, hair and make-up to create a whole look. You could own the same dress as your best friend but each of you will style it uniquely and, in this way, feel completely yourselves. That is the power and pleasure found in styling. And that's why I love showing women how to *style* their clothes, not simply wear them.

Evolving your personal style

Throughout our lives, our personal style will evolve (thank goodness!). Think about how your own style has shifted and changed. At times you may have dressed to fit in; at other times, to stand out. Age, lifestyle, body shape, size and income all influence how we choose and use clothing throughout our lives. When you look back, your clothes and style will reflect a particular time or moment.

Change is good but it's not always easy. In a fast-paced world when things move in and out of fashion from one minute to the next, style can seem like a constantly revolving door that's impossible to keep up with! But in this book, you're going to learn that regardless of your life stage, lifestyle, income status or body type, *you* get to choose how you present yourself to the world using your clothing and style.

Just as clothing has evolved over time (see Part 2), so has my teaching and styling methodology. When I started out, like most stylists at the time, I was far more specific with directions about how to dress for one's body shape, size, height or age. While there's merit in those questions, if you're familiar with my work, you'll know I no longer focus on such things. And what a blessing – my new approach teaches you so much more than that!

The old approach to styling was caught up in following 'the rules', such as what neckline we should wear for our bust size, the right length of pants with this or that shoe, or whether to add a belt or not. But too much information is confusing and limiting. Rather than increasing our choices, it narrows them, because we get too caught up in 'abiding by the rules'. Personal style is about more than a neckline or a 'flattering' cut. It's about your entire outfit from head to toe, including accessories, hair and make-up.

These days I help my clients focus more on how an outfit 'feels'. Rather than prioritising our search on finding clothes that 'suit their body shape', I help them build outfits that they feel good in – clothes that suit their personality, reflect the image they want to portray and work for their lifestyle and budget. I no longer focus on whether a client has broad shoulders or narrow shoulders, a small waist or a straight one, a round bum or a flat one. I no longer offer advice that dictates what a client should or shouldn't wear, what colour palette they should adhere to, or what brands they should buy.

If abandoning styling 'rules' is new to you, take heart – my clients say they find my approach incredibly liberating. After years of listening to my clients and responding to their unique needs I've learnt that there's no 'one size fits all' approach to personal styling. Nowadays, I teach women how to *style* outfits in a way that suits them. This book will challenge your thinking when it comes to understanding shapes, colours, feelings and movement, so you can choose an outfit every day with a greater sense of confidence. I will help you develop your unique personal expression in a way that can evolve with you over time – through all the changes and delights that life brings.

You get to choose how you *present yourself* to the world using your clothing and *style*.

How I approach personal style

Were you to review my daily outfits, you may find it hard to pick a single word to describe them. Me too! When asked to define my personal aesthetic, I struggle to sum it up in a few words. I think that's because my look is quite multifaceted – I'm a bit of a style chameleon. One day I can be super tailored, neutral and minimalist; the next, dressed in head-to-toe colour. I'm lucky, as I don't have a requirement to conform to any of the 'dress code standards' that might apply to other workplaces, so I can use clothing to express who I feel like being each and every day. My outfit is very much dictated by my mood, as well as the occasion or activity I'm attending and its crowd. Being so adaptable allows me to remain open to new ideas and creative impulses, which also helps me be a good stylist, as I bring this fresh approach to every client's wardrobe!

That said, whatever the event, purpose or occasion is that I am getting dressed for, the one word I use to help me focus my efforts is: **considered**. Regardless of what I'm wearing, where I'm wearing it to, who I'm trying to impress (beyond myself!), how I plan to move in it and whatever else I may do in it, I use this word to pull my outfit together. It's how I bring *style* to what I'm wearing and how you too can create a look that works, that is unique to you and that you feel comfortable in.

Part of my job is to help you find a way to express your individuality, so it might seem contradictory to suggest a single word to focus your efforts around. On one hand I agree, and later I'll get you to determine a fuller set of words that can help define your unique look. But this principle sits beneath them all and is the driving force behind them. It's as close as I might get to any kind of 'rule' I bring to the practice of styling – a guideline that's beyond any individual aesthetic choice. I use this word to ensure that each and every outfit I pull together is styled, no matter what feeling or visual I'm going for. As such, it applies to everyone interested in creating their own personal style, no matter what that is. When pulling together an outfit, I always keep this top of mind.

Irrespective of the look you're going for, if you have given serious *consideration* to the elements you're bringing together, they will have a particular energy – a synergy – that will bind them. It's about being intentional with your style decisions by bringing them back to a purpose, or a feeling, or to follow a simple plan. Throughout this book I will give you an array of techniques that you can apply to help bring such intentionality to your outfit planning. This is the essence of personal style.

How does 'considered' look?

If you follow me on social media or have worked with me, you'll know that a graphic t-shirt is a signature look of mine. Making this available to my clients seemed a natural evolution of my brand and I'm excited to do more in the future. I live in the heart of Melbourne city, so a very urban environment with good walkability and highly changeable weather. Depending on my day, which can range from working with a client in their home or out shopping, to going to a basketball game, to heading to the movies with my husband, I will often select one of my favourite graphic tees as my starting point, and style it in different ways. Regardless of the occasion or my mood, and the very different looks across my outfits, my decisions are thoughtful – considered – and the final result, styled.

Same piece, styled three ways

Let me explain how I style the same graphic tee in three different ways, selecting each element of my outfit carefully. I think about each item individually and how it will work across the look to create interest – either by generating coherence or contrast through small details. The styling of these three outfits does not hinge on the individual items themselves, be that the style of jeans, the length of the jacket, the height of the heel, the fit of the t-shirt, the brand of the handbag or the cost of the blazer. Each outfit comes down to thoughtful combinations worn together to make a cohesive outfit. Instinctively we respond to that – we can 'sense' when a look is styled but up to now you may not have had the language or awareness to understand why. In this book, you're going to learn how.

Going to work ↗

This look needs to be professional in a creative way, to project my work as a stylist, but also be practical and comfortable, as my job typically involves a lot of walking and moving around as we shop. My leopard slingbacks are refined in shape and interesting in texture, and the kitten heel is comfortable to wear. The black wide-leg jeans with a statement cuff are unique and modern, and the length helps to highlight my fabulous shoes. I purposely selected the brown blazer to both complement the tones in the leopard heels and pick up the brown in the t-shirt. The blazer exudes professionalism and adds polish to the denim and graphic tee. I use my accessories to add splashes of fun and colour, to showcase my creative side. The red bag and knit strategically highlight the small red detail in the tee, and the black jeans help to ground the contrasting colours and textures in the outfit.

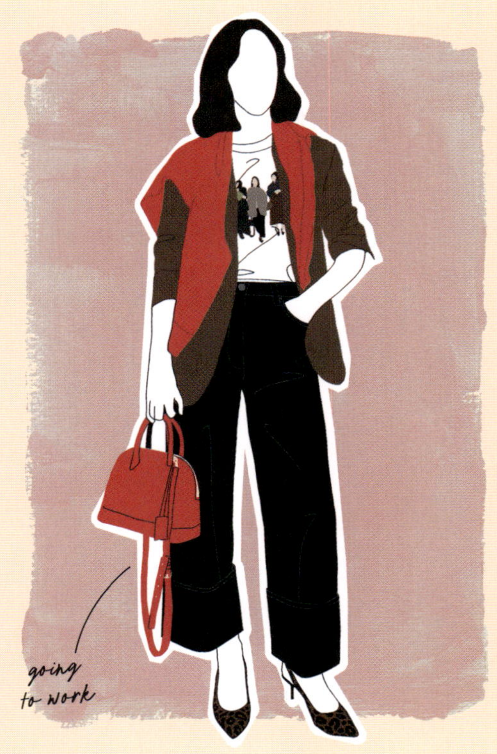
going to work

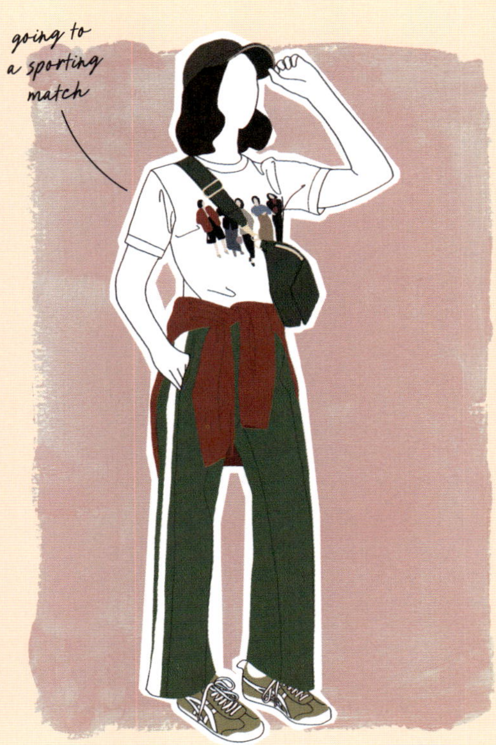
going to a sporting match

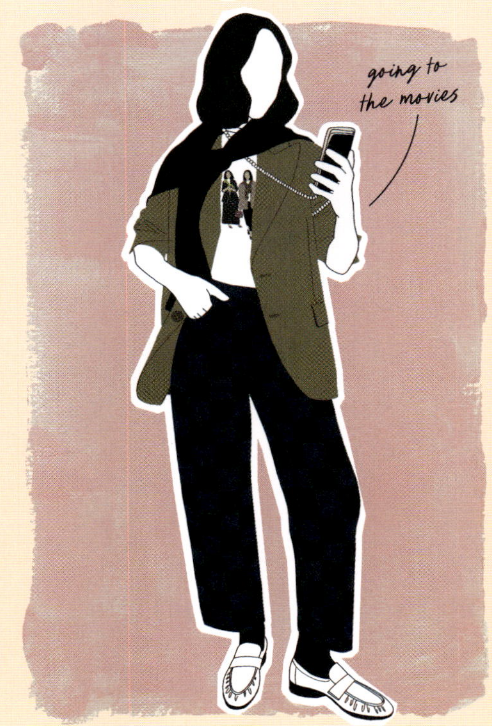
going to the movies

Going to a sporting match ↖

Whether indoors or outdoors, going to a game is a fun, festive and physical occasion, and even as a spectator it requires a degree of 'sportiness'. Yet, being a public outing, your stay-at-home trackie daks won't cut it here. Instead, I've chosen elevated green sweatpants. Their contrasting white racer stripe adds a luxe, sporty element while still feeling stylish and casual. The rust sweater ties in with the colour pops of deep orange in the graphic tee and tying it around my waist adds some definition and visual interest considering I'm not wearing a jacket. My green crossbody bag not only complements my green pants but adds further shape, cutting a diagonal across my centre. Its gold hardware is also highlighted in my gold sneakers, both adding a touch of glam in a fun and intentional way. The neutral cap not only adds to my sporty aesthetic, but also works tonally with the rest of the outfit (and covers my unwashed hair!).

Going to the movies ↙

Going on a date with my husband to the movies I want to look cute and stylish but feel relaxed. Jeans are the perfect candidate for such outings, adding a relaxed but cool vibe, especially this loose style with an interesting pattern. A blazer adds my non-negotiable (some might say 'signature') polish, and I choose an olive green one instead of navy to avoid looking like I'm in a suit. I instead wear a dark navy knit over my shoulders and wear the same shade of socks, not only for warmth but to visually complement the shade of denim. The olive blazer strategically brings out the similar hues in my t-shirt. I could have opted for a low heel in a contrasting colour with socks but in this case, I've chosen white loafers for comfort. The pearl phone chain adds a subtle connection to the shoes both in colour and uptown style.

In each outfit, the colours in my graphic tee helped me to *consider* what colours I chose from my wardrobe. When choosing these, I *considered* what was appropriate for the activity. And knowing the activity helped me to create a *considered*, intentional and suitably stylish look.

Start with your wardrobe purpose

Before we can start styling our outfits, we must consider our starting point – the clothes and accessories in our wardrobe. At this point many stylists will advise you to conduct a 'wardrobe review' then curate a 'capsule wardrobe'. We'll revisit these ideas in more detail later but let me say briefly that in its most basic form, I'm not a fan of the capsule. Controversial, perhaps! But I think our clothing choices are far more nuanced than that.

That's why I suggest we start by determining our **wardrobe purpose**. We all buy and wear clothes but how often do we consider the purpose we need them to serve each day? It's easy to get caught up in the excitement of clothes shopping and forget about the practicalities. How often have you purchased something that you 'had to have' because it was so unique, was on sale or looked great on someone else, or you loved the colour, only for it to sit in your wardrobe because you didn't have anywhere to wear it?

Think of those items in your wardrobe that still have the tags on them, or that you've never worn but can't bear to throw out. Is it the patterned silk kaftan you bought while on summer holidays in Europe, which, sadly, makes no sense in your everyday city life? Perhaps it's the corporate suit you spent big dollars on for a job interview – although you landed the job, it never gets worn because the office dress code is far more casual. Or is it that designer jacket you bought at an irresistible discount – beautifully crafted with statement shoulders and intricate beading but incompatible with your small-country-town life?

This is an example of the 'Pareto principle', or 80/20 rule, which suggests that 80 per cent of results come from just 20 per cent input. Applying this concept to our wardrobes, we see that 80 per cent of the time we wear just 20 per cent of our clothes, leaving most of them barely touched. Having a closet filled with clothes that don't serve a purpose can feel overwhelming and even demoralising – they become a daily reminder of how much money we have spent, the size we used to be or the life we used to live.

No one needs to carry that weight, so let's find ways to shed it. Imagine clearing that space – the clutter, the confusion and the mental noise – and instead having a wardrobe of clothes that reflects the person you are today and holds room for the person you want to be tomorrow. At this point, a standard 'wardrobe review' would have you analyse your wardrobe and ditch anything you're not wearing. But I don't want you to get rid of any clothes just yet. By the end of this book, you may well be making very good use of them.

Let me show you how to create a highly functional and hard-working **80/20 wardrobe** – where you'll use 80 per cent of your wardrobe almost all the time and even put the lazy 20 per cent to use. Our first step is to think about our wardrobe (and any new pieces we introduce into it) in a more logical, pragmatic and thoughtful way – by reviewing each item of clothing in light of your wardrobe purpose. Once you've done this, you'll easily see why most of it is being worn so rarely. Perhaps your closet is filled with clothes from the previous decade – a corporate wardrobe and career you've retired from. Perhaps, since you love fashion, you're an impulse shopper, so you've ended up with a mismatched wardrobe of fabulous 'one-offs' but no staples to pull an outfit together. Or are you simply someone who shops for the life you'd like to live rather than the one you actually have, leaving you a mere handful of practical things to wear over and over again?

Knowing your wardrobe purpose makes you a better shopper. It gives you a process that leads you to buy what your wardrobe and lifestyle need, rather than things you might wear once, twice or never. You'll find yourself buying clothes with greater intention and enjoying a much higher rate of success. No longer will you have a wardrobe full of clothes but nothing to wear! Instead, you'll have a wardrobe of clothes that you love and wear often, providing great value for money. The result is a highly functioning wardrobe that works, ensures low cost-per-wear and can be adapted to suit all aspects of our lives.

A look at my wardrobe purpose

Determining your wardrobe purpose is a straightforward activity. Essentially, you want to figure out what you spend most of your time doing, to which you'll allocate most of your wardrobe (80 per cent), and then allocate the remaining 20 per cent to any activities and clothes that are important but occur less frequently. That way you can have a wardrobe full of clothes that match your everyday reality and lifestyle.

To help you determine your wardrobe purpose, it's important to ask yourself one very simple question. It's a question I ask clients every single day and one I ask myself too.

'Where will you wear it?'

It's common for my clients to get very excited about the prospect of new clothes when we're shopping together. All these lovely new things to touch and feel, all so shiny and new, and very tempting! I watch a client's eyes divert to a beautiful one-shoulder summer dress with the most divine floral print. They love it. They want it. But do they *really* need it?

At this point I ask: '*Where will you wear it?*' With this question I'm asking clients to determine the relevance of the item to their current lifestyle; to think about its functionality and purpose in their lives *today* – not in the life they wish they had, or that they used to have. I'm asking them: 'What does your life look like *right now*, what purpose does your wardrobe serve, and does this item fit that purpose?'

Let's review my own wardrobe in these terms.

My 80 per cent 'everyday' wardrobe

It's fair to say that work is my main priority and something that takes up much of my day, Monday to Saturday. Most of that time is spent on my feet, in public, so I need to dress in a way that is stylish, elevated and modern yet practical. This remains true, even when working from home, although there I can be a little more casual and comfortable. I'm also fortunate that, living in the heart of a big city, my everyday work style overlaps with and merges into my non-work wardrobe. What I wear to work, I can also wear to a restaurant or a comedy show.

When I examine my lifestyle and my wardrobe purpose, it's obvious that for me, my work and social life are the most demanding – they are my 80 per cent. This understanding allows me to make objective decisions when contemplating a purchase; that is, if I can wear it to work and a social event, it fits my wardrobe purpose. Since work is the main purpose of my wardrobe, when I go shopping, work-friendly options are my biggest focus. So, when I'm looking to add something new, I ask myself, 'Would I wear this to work?' If I can wear it to work, I can generally wear it socially too. I might choose different shoes or a different handbag, but the core outfit is the same.

Asking 'Where will I wear it?' also helps me with my budget. In fashion, we love a little calculation called 'cost-per-wear' and use it to determine the value we'll get from a purchase by dividing its purchase price by the number of times we'll wear it. A school uniform would have a low cost-per-wear, since it's not too expensive to start with, say $100 for a tunic that will be worn a few days a week for several years. At $100 divided by, say, 600 days, that gives us a cost-per-wear of just 17 cents.

I use this calculation to help me determine what I'm happy to spend on a new purchase. If I'm going to wear an item a lot, aka, 80 per cent of the time, then its cost-per-wear drops. If it's something I'll wear to work every week, that complements my wardrobe and feels like me, then I'll consider spending more money on it. On the other hand, if I'm only ever going to wear it a few times a year, I'll re-evaluate.

I love suiting but not the traditional corporate style. Modern suiting has become part of our everyday lives, well beyond the boardroom. We now wear suits with sneakers, with t-shirts, in wool and linen, in black and yellow. Suits are something I find handy to throw on when I'm having one of those 'I have nothing to wear' kind of days or when, despite having a wardrobe of clothes I love, the creative juices aren't flowing. A suit is a quick and easy choice that feels polished, put together and considered.

I also love the versatility a suit brings to my wardrobe. I can wear the jacket and pants separately with other pieces, and by mixing and matching, I can achieve a range of different outfit combinations that always keep my look fresh and interesting. For example, for work, I can style a suit with a striped cotton shirt, pointed-toe slingback kitten heels and a smart handbag. For lunch, I could style the suit pants with the same shirt worn unbuttoned over a graphic tee and wear a more casual loafer shoe and crossbody bag. For a fashion event, I might decide to wear the full suit with a sheer top and lace bra and add silver heels and a statement clutch. For a weekend catch-up with the family, I'd wear the jacket with some modern jeans and ballet flats, a jumper over my shoulders and a canvas tote.

For me, a suit serves my wardrobe purpose 80 per cent of the time. It's high on functionality, strong on style and has a low cost-per-wear, meaning it's great value for money overall.

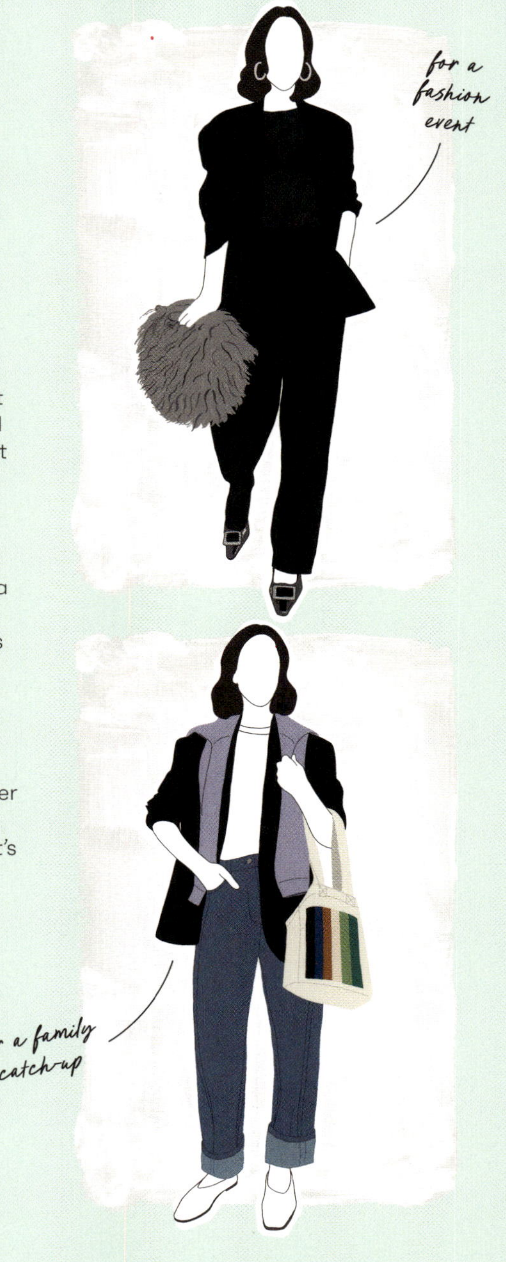

My 20 per cent 'occasional' wardrobe

So, what about the other 20 per cent? Well, it's made up of a few categories of clothing that I need for things I do often enough to justify giving them space in my wardrobe but not so frequently that they should take up too much room. As you can see, the purpose served by the 20 per cent is important – what I wear every now and then is still a functioning part of my wardrobe that I rely on when the time is right. Although rarely used, these pieces still align with my personal style, reflect my **style personality** (more on this in the next chapter) and make me feel good when I wear them. Let's take a closer look at what's in my 20 per cent wardrobe so you can see what I mean.

Resortwear

My husband and I like to go on holidays to hot places like Queensland. Being from Melbourne, I don't really have the need for 'resort-style' clothing like silk pants, linen sets, strappy sandals or sundresses, but over time I've built up a great capsule wardrobe of these pieces for our getaways. This means I can pack the same items every trip, allowing me to repeat outfits and feel relaxed (and cool!) in the destination climate. This section of my wardrobe serves a small purpose. Knowing this helps me resist the urge to buy too many beautiful new strapless silk maxi-dresses each time summer comes around.

Athleisure

I do Pilates twice a week and occasionally go for long walks. I don't particularly care about being in the 'latest' activewear, so I wear what I own, on high rotation. I don't need three drawers full of leggings and crop tops (okay, I don't really need any crop tops!), so when I buy new activewear it's usually to replace something that's had its day. My activewear takes up minimal space, for minimal wear. And while I love being at home, I'm not really a homebody. For weeknights and the odd Sunday at home relaxing or making content, all I need is one pair of tracksuit pants, a couple of jumpers and a cashmere lounge set.

Formalwear

At this stage of my life, I don't have many formal occasions to attend – celebrations like weddings and engagement parties, or annual events like charity balls or going to the races. If I do have something pop up, I'll either re-wear something I already have and love, or hire an outfit for the occasion.

A 20 per cent item – the sneaker

I have deliberately chosen a provocative item as my 20 per cent example to show you that each person's wardrobe is different. For so many people, sneakers have become a go-to shoe of choice and therefore part of their 80 per cent wardrobe. With more workplaces having casual dress codes, sneakers are now appropriate to wear to work, then on to dinner or the theatre afterwards and many women relish their newfound heel-free freedom.

I too joined the sneaker chorus for a while and started wearing them instead of my much-loved (and signature) pointed-toe kitten heels or ankle boots. But despite their rise in popularity, I soon realised they were too casual for my taste. I returned to wearing what I call 'elevated' flat shoes, for which I have three alternatives: ballet flats (never thought I'd say that!), loafers and strappy sandals. These shoe styles feel more me – more polished, unique and modern.

Because they don't feel right for me, sneakers only fulfil a 20 per cent purpose in my wardrobe. I wear them for the occasional casual Sunday catch-up at a friend's house or a weekend away. I wear the pairs I already own and don't feel the need to buy another pair.

Defining my wardrobe purpose

Shortly, you'll complete a two-step activity to define your wardrobe purpose. Here is an example of mine. By reviewing my clothes in light of my lifestyle (my wardrobe purpose) – where I wear them, why, when and how often – I easily identified whether an item belonged in my 80 per cent 'everyday' wardrobe or my 20 per cent 'occasional' wardrobe.

Sally's wardrobe purpose

Item	Where, why?	When, how often?	80 or 20 per cent?
activewear	training	year-round, twice a week	20 per cent
ankle boots	work, social	year-round, most days and nights	80 per cent
ballet flats	work, social	year-round, most days and nights	80 per cent
blazers	work, social	year-round, most days and nights	80 per cent
cashmere jumpers	work, social	all seasons except summer, most days and nights	80 per cent
casual skirts/dresses	daytime casual weekends	rarely, summer only	20 per cent
chunky jumpers	work, social	winter only, most days and nights	20 per cent
coats	work, social	winter only, most days and nights	20 per cent
formal dresses	events	very rarely	20 per cent
jeans	work, social	year-round, most days and nights	80 per cent
kitten heels	work, social	year-round though less often in winter, most days and nights	80 per cent
knee-high boots	work, social	winter only, most days and nights	20 per cent
linen, linen sets	summer, holidays	rarely, holidays only	20 per cent
loafers	work, social	year-round, most days and nights	80 per cent
shorts	daytime casual weekends	rarely, summer only	20 per cent
smart dresses	work, social	year-round, most days and nights	80 per cent
sneakers	casual	year-round, Sundays only	20 per cent
suits	work, social	year-round, most days and nights	80 per cent
swimwear	summer, holidays	rarely, holidays only	20 per cent
tailored pants	work, social	year-round, most days and nights	80 per cent
tracksuit pants	lounging, home only	rarely	20 per cent
t-shirts	work, social	year-round, most days and nights	80 per cent

Sally's 80/20 wardrobe

80 per cent 'everyday' wardrobe	20 per cent 'occasional' wardrobe
ankle boots	activewear
ballet flats	casual skirts/dresses
blazers	chunky jumpers
cashmere jumpers	coats
jeans	formal dresses
kitten heels	knee-high boots
loafers	linen, linen sets
smart dresses	shorts
suits	sneakers
tailored pants	swimwear
t-shirts	tracksuit pants

Activity: Determine your wardrobe purpose

What you need:
pen and paper

So now it's time to determine *your* wardrobe purpose. In this activity you'll review each item in your wardrobe against your lifestyle to ultimately define your 80/20 wardrobe. Doing this was somewhat easy for me, since my work and social-life wardrobes overlap. Your wardrobe purpose will naturally look different from mine as it will reflect how your clothes work in with your daily life. To get the most from this activity you should review everything – include shoes, bags, hats, formalwear, holiday clothes, loungewear and activewear. You will feel an amazing sense of clarity once you complete this, so are you ready? Let's get started.

1. Create a four-column table with the following headings: 1) Item, 2) Where/why?, 3) When/how often?, 4) 80 or 20 per cent?

2. Start by listing all the items currently in your wardrobe. Rather than listing each item individually, try to group them into like-for-like items. For me 'jeans' is enough but you might want to distinguish between 'casual jeans' and 'dress jeans' if they have a different purpose in your wardrobe.

3. Think about *where* and *why* you wear these. Is it for work or social, casually or formally, daytime or nighttime? Use these categories if they're helpful or come up with some of your own.

4. Now, think about *how often* you wear these. Is it year-round or only for a short season, every day or for a specific activity, and if so, how regularly?

5. Finally, review the previous three columns. We often have a skewed idea of how important a piece of clothing is but reviewing each piece in this way will make clear how often you really use it. With this information at hand, decide whether it belongs in your 80 per cent or your 20 per cent wardrobe.

6. Create a new table of two columns to reveal your 80/20 wardrobe.

Knowing your wardrobe purpose will make you a *better shopper*.

The 80/20 wardrobe in action

Once you've completed this activity it's easy to see the reality of where and when you use your clothes. At this point you may be tempted to start tossing clothes out or rushing out to buy new ones. (Why did I have so many summer dresses, I asked myself at this point!) But don't be too hasty. Unless they're truly falling apart and unable to be mended, we may find a use for them yet – this is only the first chapter, and we still have much to work through! In the coming pages you will learn how to repurpose your wardrobe, create new outfit combinations and uncover your personal style. This will allow you to wear more of what you own more often and dress more confidently.

Eventually, with all those tools in hand you will be ready to make changes to your wardrobe. At that point, the 80/20 approach will help you shop with greater clarity. You'll stop spending money on things you don't need and never wear and instead have a wardrobe full of clothes you love that you wear on repeat.

Keeping the 80/20 theory in mind, as you do a wardrobe clean-out and before you buy, ask yourself these questions:

1. When/where will I wear it?

2. What purpose will this serve in my wardrobe?

3. How often will I wear it?

4. Do I have something similar that achieves the same outcome?

On the following pages, we'll take a look at how this works for some of my clients.

Lin's wardrobe purpose

Lin works full-time in a hospital where she wears a uniform of scrubs. She is married with two young children, so most weekends are spent at kids' sports and parties, going on bike rides and at weekly park catch-ups with other local families. Lin's social activities include the occasional casual family restaurant or a long walk and coffee with a friend. She goes to the horseraces once a year and attends a wedding or engagement party every now and then. When not working, Lin spends a lot of time at home with the children. She is a homebody at heart and is most happy cooking, watching movies and being in the garden. She lives in a cool climate where temperatures occasionally reach the high 20s in summer.

In determining her wardrobe purpose, Lin sees that, outside work, 80 per cent of her time is spent on daytime socialising and casual family-friendly evenings. She also lives in a cool climate. This means that most of her personal wardrobe should be allocated to jeans, tops she can layer for warmth including casual jackets, and practical shoes like sneakers and ankle boots. With only a few months of the year warm enough, she only needs a few summer items. When the yearly races come around, instead of buying a new dress, Lin might wear something she already has but update it with new accessories, or even hire a dress, since it's such a rare occasion. Being clear on her wardrobe purpose means that even when Lin is taken by, say, a pair of sparkly jewelled satin pumps in the store window, she can say 'no thanks' despite the fact that they are half-price.

Lin's 80/20 wardrobe

80 per cent 'everyday' wardrobe
boots, casual jackets, fleecy jumpers, jeans, knitwear, long-sleeve tops, sneakers, t-shirts.

20 per cent 'occasional' wardrobe
dressy top, formal dress, high heels, sandals, shorts, summer dress.

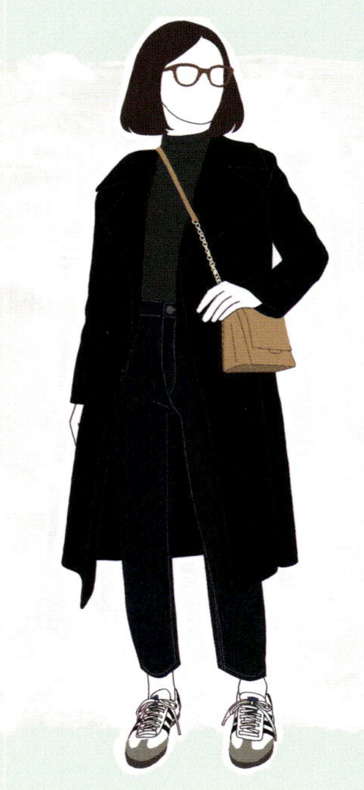

Marnie's wardrobe purpose

Marnie is a stay-at-home mum living in a seaside town where the climate is warm and humid most of the year. Her days revolve around school drop-off and pick-up, running errands, doing housework and shopping for groceries. After school, there is a lot of driving the kids from activity to activity. Twice a week Marnie takes her mum out for lunch to a local suburban café. Marnie and her partner go out on date nights every month, and she enjoys after-hours social activities with other school mums.

In reviewing her wardrobe purpose, Marnie sees that her clothing priorities are ones that suit her town's casual vibe, beachside location and warm weather. She barely wears the beautiful winter coat she bought in London, so, despite new drops being featured across her social media feed throughout winter, she is able to say no to buying any more. When summer rolls around and her feed updates to easy-wear, low-maintenance summer dresses, it's a different story. With all her day-to-day running around, refreshing her selection of dresses makes sense, as they are the perfect 'throw on and go' item for her. She can wear them with Birkenstocks for the school run, dress them up with nice sandals to take her mum out for lunch, and pair them with a dressier heel and handbag for a night out with the school mums.

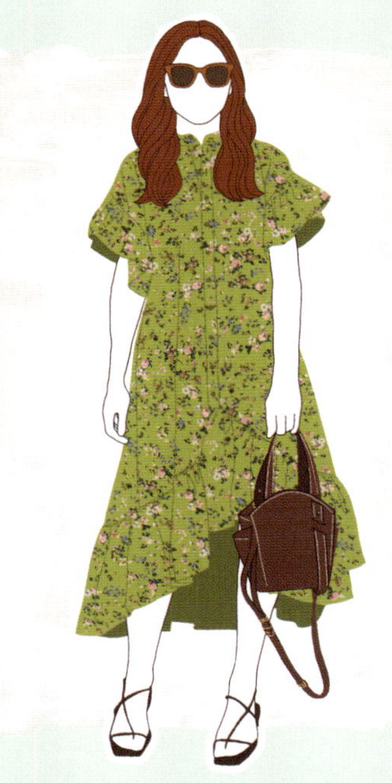

Marnie's 80/20 wardrobe

80 per cent 'everyday' wardrobe
active wear, casual bag, linen pants, sandals, shorts, sneakers, summer dresses, swimwear, tank tops, t-shirts.

20 per cent 'occasional' wardrobe
ankle boots, coat, dress heels, dressy tops, evening bag, jeans, linen blazer.

Same lifestyle, different style

Although Marnie and Lin appear to have similar lifestyles, both being busy mums of young families, their 80/20 wardrobes look very different because of their wardrobe purpose, their climate and, most importantly, their unique style personality – which we'll explore in the next chapter. Following that we will create a modular wardrobe that suits all occasions and moods, challenge your thinking when it comes to your body shape, empower you to use social media for good, uncover tips and tricks for keeping your wardrobe fresh, learn how to pack with style and how to tweak an outfit to look just right. All these tools will help you build the confidence you deserve when getting dressed. I can't wait for you to learn more!

When you look back, your clothes and style will reflect a particular *time* or *moment*.

2. DEFINE YOUR STYLE PERSONALITY

Now that we've determined your wardrobe purpose and you have a clearer idea of all the items you own, we move into the next exciting phase. This will help you decide which pieces to hold onto and how to repurpose others. In this chapter you'll learn to describe your **style personality**. It's not a matter of fashion (though it can tie into that) but a matter of style. Let me explain . . .

Your style personality won't change as often as fashion does but there is certainly room for it to evolve and grow with you as you change throughout your life. Fashion, on the other hand, is a fast-paced beast, shifting rapidly from season to season (some might say week to week). The wide range of choice we see in stores and online can be intimidating and confusing. These days, online shopping allows us to fill our closets with the click of a button, to express ship from anywhere in the world, to buy now, pay later. Together with the wide range of local designer labels and stores, fashion meets a broad range of needs, from inclusive sizing, adaptive clothing, ethical and sustainable fashion to fast fashion and reselling. And while this greater choice is exhilarating, it can also lead to more uncertainty and tougher decisions.

The answer to navigating this confidently is unearthing our style personality. This is what underpins and differentiates our personal style from others. It is an instinctual and fundamental part of our style DNA, evident in every outfit we wear. It's what makes us feel like ourselves in some clothing and an imposter in others. Identifying and determining our style personality will help us be better shoppers, better decision-makers, better self-stylers and better at using clothes to embody the person we want to be. It's like having your own stylist in your pocket!

In this chapter, to help you identify your own style personality, we're going to do a few more activities. You've already determined your wardrobe purpose, and now you're going to start shopping for clothes with a new mindset. Knowing your wardrobe purpose and style personality will help you be more disciplined in your spending and more decisive in your style choices, because they will all align.

Knowing your style

Many people I work with feel very under-confident in their style. 'I don't have any style, Sally!' they say. 'That's why I've come to you!'

This is blatantly untrue. They – like me, and you, and everyone else on this planet! – have been developing their style from the time they could see. Nevertheless, there are ways we can continue to develop our style until we feel confident with it. Let's take a look.

Develop your artistic eye

Do you recall me leaving teaching for my six-month solo trip around the world? I was craving inspiration. Travel is a fabulous way to soak up artistic ways of seeing and being. From galleries to monuments to everyday street fashion, being away from your daily life is a balm for the soul and a rich way to fill your creative cup. Simply as I walked down Fifth Avenue, I saw an incredibly diverse range of communities, each with their own distinct style and culture. Not to mention the inspiration I gained from travelling across Europe and the UK.

Because of the experiences I had then, I know how vital travel is to sustain my creativity. Instinctively, I think most of us are aware of that, which is why Australians are so renowned for being world travellers. These days we're lucky enough to be able to do it from home too, as we scroll through social media, though nothing beats soaking up a new place with all your senses. (And yes, if you're wondering, later I dedicate a whole chapter to how we can pack and still look stylish while doing so – hold on tight!).

While we don't always have the time, budget or ability to travel abroad to get this hit of creative input, we *can* intentionally seek out inspiration in our very own backyards: each weekend can be an opportunity to explore a different neighbourhood or scene. Visiting a variety of retailers, not just clothing stores but others too, perhaps jewellery and furniture stores, or markets and vintage stores, or designer and artisan galleries, can be incredibly rewarding. It also helps you develop your eye if you notice what you are drawn to. What makes you curious or gives you a little thrill? What sticks in your memory when the day is over? This understanding of what you naturally gravitate towards can inspire the development of your style personality through mixing and matching different elements that you love.

Recognise your personal influences

I was fortunate enough to have a mother who encouraged me in such explorations of style, and with it, influenced my love of clothing and personal dress. Mum was always very well dressed herself – not in a 'high fashion' kind of way but in a considered way. She always complemented her outfits with a statement necklace or scarf, knew how to pair colours for aesthetic appeal, and always had an appreciation for what was considered stylish at any given time in her life.

Like many women of her generation, I don't think she spent a lot of money on clothes but she always seemed to have plenty of them! She would dress my sister and me beautifully, making a lot of our clothes when we were younger (she was very creative, an art teacher). As we grew older, she didn't particularly like clothes shopping and she loved a bargain, so she'd take us to local markets and second-hand stalls rather than shopping centres or department stores. She'd let my sister and me rifle through the clothes while she looked at the plants, ceramics, tea towels, picture frames . . . anything but clothes! In this way, we ended up with a fairly unconventional wardrobe, certainly not what you'd describe as mainstream, and we often looked a bit different from everyone else.

Reflecting on my approach to style, I can see that my mother nurtured this in me from a young age. She instilled me with an interest in and appreciation of personal style, then 'set me free' to explore, discover, succeed and fail with clothing all by myself. Although my mother didn't share my love of shopping, she did impress on me the value of an individual aesthetic and developing one's unique personal style.

Travel is a *fabulous* way to soak up artistic ways of seeing and being.

Activity: Consider your influences

What you need:
pen and paper

Thinking about who in your life (past or present) inspires you with what they wear may help reveal your style preferences. Actively seeking out external influences can help fine-tune your artistic eye and shape the way you dress. Being an active observer helps you notice what you do and don't like. Perhaps it's admiring the way your fellow commuter always matches his bag, belt and shoes. Perhaps it's gathering your friends for a clothes swap party. Maybe it's learning more about cultural periods from your friend the art teacher. Or perhaps it's following who they follow on social media. Spend some time reflecting on these questions:

1. Who in your childhood did you admire creatively – for the way they dressed or how they showed up creatively? What places did you enjoy for how they were styled?

2. How did being around them/it make you feel?

3. What was it about what they wore, what you did or how it was presented that you liked? Lean into your senses to help you with this – think about colours, shapes, sounds, smells, touch, taste.

4. Is there someone (or some place) in your life today who evokes a similar response? Describe them/it.

5. What similarities across these people and places are you drawn to? Are there certain colours, textures, sounds, smells or feelings that pop up time and time again?

6. Would you like to bring some of those elements into your own style? How might you do this?

Take inspiration from social media

One of the biggest changes I've seen in my clients over the years is their use of social media to help them get inspired by fashion. When I work with a new client for the first time, I ask them to share images of looks or styles they love. From these images, I can immediately tell what look the client wants to achieve and their personal style preferences.

It's also a useful way to separate what we genuinely like from what we think we *should* like. I've worked with women who tell me that they want to introduce more colour into their wardrobes but then I look at their inspiration images and there's no colour. They're not actually drawn to colour, and that's why they don't wear it. But because they don't wear it, they think they should!

Visuals help us formulate ideas about how to put together outfits or what styles we feel drawn to and can help us start to narrow down and identify what our own personal style is. They are a powerful tool.

Platforms like Pinterest, Instagram, TikTok, Facebook, blogs, newsletters and fashion and retail sites provide us with ideas to experiment with. They can help us think outside the box when it comes to styling and expose us to new ways of wearing what we already own. If we're feeling confused, frustrated or uninspired with our own wardrobes, we can turn to these for endless inspiration. Thanks to social media, anyone, anywhere in the world, can share their personal style and you and I can benefit from it.

Who to follow

Perhaps you're thinking that it won't be *your* style personality if it draws too much from other people. Let me reassure you: there is absolutely nothing wrong with being inspired by other people's style and copying elements of their outfits. I do it all the time. We can't all reinvent the wheel (that's what fashion designers and stylists are for!) so why not use the available tools to help you shop and get dressed with greater ease and purpose?

When deciding who to follow, I have three simple tips. Follow creators:

1. whose style you admire

2. who inspire you to style your wardrobe in new ways

3. who make you feel more confident.

This doesn't mean you should only follow people who look like you, have the same shape or body size as you, or are the same age as you. I feel that's irrelevant: style is style, no matter who's wearing it, and you don't have to look like someone to be inspired by them. I draw inspiration from a wide variety of women – and men! – on social media. Follow anyone who inspires you. You might follow person A because their style personality resonates with yours, even though they're a completely different body shape. You follow person B because they wear a lot of brands you like, and even though their seasons are opposite you can shop these brands out of season and on sale. Perhaps person C wears clothes that are far beyond your own budget but they inspire you to style your existing wardrobe in new ways.

I also offer style inspiration to my online community as well as my clients using social media: providing ideas on how to style the pieces you already own in new ways, encouraging you to try something new regardless of your age, and suggesting pieces you can replicate with brands that suit your own budget.

Get inspired

If you haven't already used the internet or some form of social media to seek style inspiration, now is the time to start! I cannot stress enough how valuable these are in helping you to define your personal style.

Scrolling for inspiration can be a tedious task but capturing these visual references as you spot them will help future you! Here the social media algorithm works to our benefit. The algorithm learns our behaviours and when we engage with the accounts we like (i.e. like a post, comment, save or share with our friends), we'll be targeted with similar accounts as we scroll our feeds, whether they're fashion and style, politics and pooches, or travel and tapas.

When you're browsing apps or websites on your phone, you'll notice certain images inspire you so much that they 'stop the scroll'. When your eyes land on them, your interest is captured in a split-second and you pause to examine them. An outfit might not speak to you from head to toe but there'll be something about the aesthetic of the pieces together and the emotions triggered that grabbed your attention. Perhaps it's the drape of the trousers, even though they're not your preferred colour, or the shape of the jacket, even though it's being worn with shoes you'd never go for.

When you find someone whose style you love, look at who they follow. This is a great way to find other accounts who create the type of content you want to see more of. Instagram and Pinterest are particularly useful platforms for this as they allow you to save preferences and will curate your feed. Their built-in algorithms will start to learn your preferences and introduce you to new content. While this is a great way to grow your connections, be mindful that it can also limit your range to specific ideas and aesthetics. On the whole, however, it's useful as over time you will notice a trend developing, which is a good indicator of your style preferences.

Visuals . . . are a *powerful* tool.

Curate your content

Use hashtags

Using hashtags and the algorithm, I have been able to curate a feed of content that inspires my personal style every day. Most creators include specific hashtags in their content for the specific purpose of being discovered. If you follow a hashtag, posts using that tag will appear in your feed without you needing to follow all the individual accounts.

Just as you would use your internet browser to search for something specific, you can use hashtags to find style accounts of people who, for example:

- are the same age as you – #50plusstyle
- live in the same city – #londonstyle
- wear the same brands – #tibifans
- share the same values – #ethicalshopping
- have a similar style personality – #minimaliststyle
- are the same size as you – #inclusivefashion.

Use your 80 per cent

Choose one of your 80 per cent wardrobe items and look it up using your platform's search function (for example: 'blazer outfit women') to find good examples of how others wear it. Look through the search results and save any images that 'stop the scroll' – anything that causes you to pause and take note.

Activity: Find your style inspiration

What you need:
your phone, laptop or computer

1. Select your chosen app or software – Google search, Instagram and/or Pinterest are all good for this.

2. Create a folder or board in which to save images, called 'style inspiration'.

3. Now, search your chosen platform and start selecting and saving any images that 'stop the scroll'.

4. Continue to do this over a period – perhaps a few weeks or if this is your first time doing it, I'd suggest saving images for a month or so before you complete the 'Style personality' activity that comes later in the chapter.

Activity: Define your wardrobe style

What you need:
pen and paper
clothing rack, bed or clear floor space
your phone camera

1. Pull out up to 10 items from your wardrobe that you wear on high rotation. When making your selections, choose only one piece from each category. For example, if you wear sneakers on high rotation and you own multiple pairs, just choose one pair. If printed dresses are your thing and you wear several of them regularly, just pull out one. Same for jeans, blazers, black pants, silk shirts . . . just choose one as your reference. Include shoes, as these are a crucial part of our personal style, but not handbags.

2. If you've got a portable rail, hang them here. If not, lay them out on your bed or floor. Take a photo on your phone.

3. Now, look at each item and select up to three words to describe it. This should not so much be a physical description of its shape, colour and material but words that describe how it makes you feel when you are wearing it and/or the image or persona it helps you project. Over the page I've provided a list of words but don't feel you must stick to them. Create a continuous list, so that by the end, for 10 items, you will end up with between thirty to ninety words. It is completely fine if you find yourself using similar words or repeating them.

4. Now, look at what you've written. Across your complete list of words, what are the three to five most common words? Circle or highlight them. These words define your current 'wardrobe style'.

Activity helper: Word list

Use this for:
- 'Define your wardrobe style' activity
- 'Determine your style personality' activity

Adventurous, Alternative, Amused, Androgynous, Artistic, Assured, Attractive, Balanced, Bold, Bright, Calm, Carefree, Capable, Casual, Cheerful, Chic, Clever, Clean, Comfortable, Complex, Confident, Considerate, Cool, Cosy, Creative, Delicate, Detailed, Distinguished, Dramatic, Dreamy, Eclectic, Edgy, Effortless, Elegant, Energetic, Expressive, Fabulous, Fearless, Feminine, Flirty, Flowy, Folksy, Fragile, Free, Fresh, Friendly, Fun, Funky, Gentle, Glam, Global, Graceful, Groovy, Grungy, Grounded, Happy, Harmonious, Imaginative, Impressive, Innovative, Intentional, Intense, Intelligent, Joyful, Laidback, Lively, Lovely, Luxurious, Masculine, Minimal, Modest, Modern, Mysterious, Natural, Neutral, Nostalgic, Optimistic, Organic, Ornate, Organised, Outdoorsy, Oversized, Pampered, Passionate, Peaceful, Playful, Polished, Powerful, Practical, Preppy, Pretty, Professional, Pure, Purposeful, Punk, Quirky, Rational, Rebellious, Refined, Relaxed, Reserved, Retro, Rugged, Sculptural, Secure, Selective, Sensible, Sensual, Serene, Sharp, Simple, Sleek, Smart, Soft, Sophisticated, Sporty, Straightforward, Streamlined, Striking, Strong, Subtle, Surprising, Tailored, Thoughtful, Timeless, Tomboy, Unburdened, Uncomplicated, Understated, Unexpected, Unique, Unstressed, Urban, Vibrant, Warm, Welcoming, Witty, Worldly.

Sally's style personality

Part of my job as a stylist is to offer myself as a teaching tool and many of you reading this book will have picked it up because you follow me on social media. So, let's use my feed as an example. If you have been following and bookmarking my posts as part of an inspiration collection, it would contain images similar to these.

Add to these the images of me wearing my 80 per cent black blazer in two different ways back on page 15, and you'll start to see a theme developing. Regardless of what I'm doing, and whether I'm dressed more casually or formally, my outfits can usually be described using similar words.

- Working with a client: *modern, polished* and *tailored*.

- Going to the movies on the weekend: *modern, creative* and *relaxed*.

- Heading out to a bar with friends: *tailored, polished, modern, creative*.

To review these looks in more detail:

- There is often juxtaposition within the outfit, such as a *tailored* blazer with a casual pant, a sporty graphic t-shirt with a tailored trouser or *modern* jeans with a feminine heel.

- There is a contrast between minimalist, *polished* looks featuring neutral colours and bold, colourful and *creative* outfits.

- The look is always *modern* and contemporary, the silhouette balanced, and every element is considered to create a *polished* harmonious look.

Using the activities in this chapter, I found some commonalities across each of my looks, despite their variety. From this I was able to select four words that comfortably describe my style.

My style personality: *tailored, polished, modern, creative.*

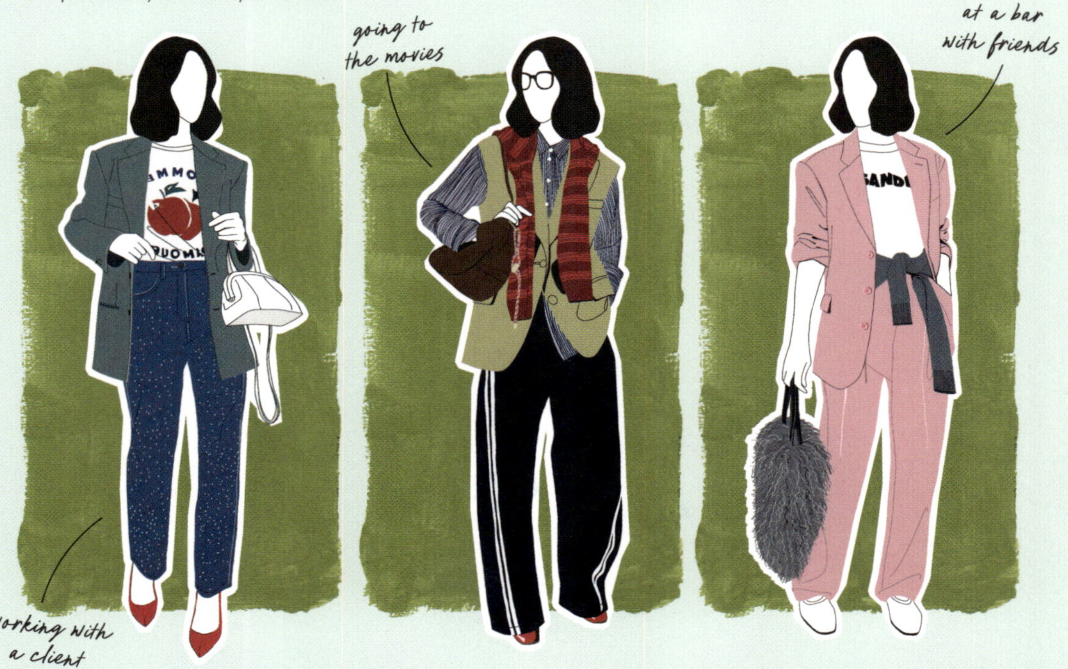

Activity: Determine your style personality

pen and paper

from the previous activities, your:

- 'style inspiration' images
- 'wardrobe style' words

For this activity you're going to try to be really honest and somewhat ruthless with yourself. I promise it won't hurt!

1. With your 'style inspiration' images and 'wardrobe style' words handy, create a new board/folder called 'My style personality'.

2. Now, assess each of your style inspiration images and ask yourself, 'Does this reflect at least one of my words?' If it does, move it across to your new 'My style personality' board/folder. If it doesn't, delete it.

3. When you're finished, turn to your new 'My style personality' board/folder. Using a piece of paper or a notes app on your phone, start to write down any similarities you see across the images. This can be in point form or paragraphs. Ask yourself:

    - What do the images have in common?

    - What do you like about them?

    - Are there any words you would use to describe the images as a collective?

    - What feelings or emotions do these outfits evoke?

    - Sometimes it helps to think in opposites: can you describe what these images do *not* portray?

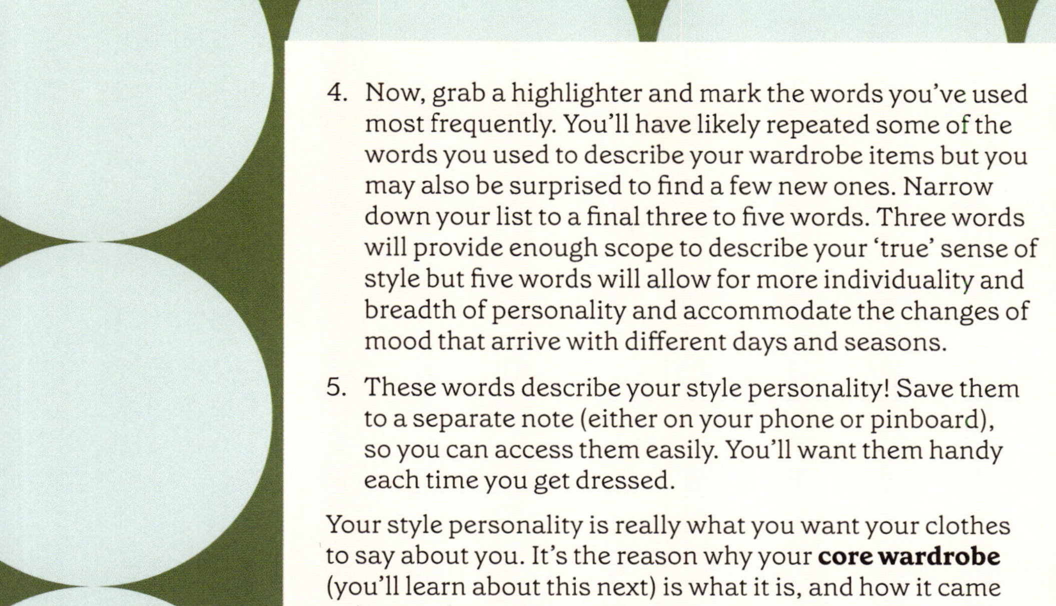

4. Now, grab a highlighter and mark the words you've used most frequently. You'll have likely repeated some of the words you used to describe your wardrobe items but you may also be surprised to find a few new ones. Narrow down your list to a final three to five words. Three words will provide enough scope to describe your 'true' sense of style but five words will allow for more individuality and breadth of personality and accommodate the changes of mood that arrive with different days and seasons.

5. These words describe your style personality! Save them to a separate note (either on your phone or pinboard), so you can access them easily. You'll want them handy each time you get dressed.

Your style personality is really what you want your clothes to say about you. It's the reason why your **core wardrobe** (you'll learn about this next) is what it is, and how it came to be. It's the reason you feel great in certain outfits and not so great in others. Unlike your wardrobe purpose, your style personality is likely to stay the same throughout your life, give or take a few tweaks here and there.

Knowing what's *not* you

Articulating your style personality will not only help you better understand your personal style – it will also help you identify what it is *not*.

When you wear something that does not align with your style personality, it will feel off. You might not be able to put your finger on exactly *what* but something doesn't feel right. You might spend your day fidgeting with or adjusting your clothes, slumping your shoulders, sucking in your stomach or even not leaving your house or desk. I'm sure, like me, you can recall a time when you've done this because you were wearing something that didn't feel great.

To avoid wearing an outfit that does not align with you, check your outfit against the words you identified to describe your style personality. Are they reflected in the clothes and accessories you are trying on? If something feels 'off' or 'not quite right', describe the outfit in front of you. Do the words you use align with your style personality? What words don't fit? Try to call them out by being really specific.

For example, if I am dressing for work, I might choose a camel blazer, a white cotton shirt, black jeans, black loafers and a cream handbag.

Words I use to describe this outfit: *tailored, polished, timeless.*

As a reminder, my style personality: *tailored, polished, modern, creative.*

Reviewing my outfit against my style personality, I can see the outfit feels too timeless, which for me means that it feels too predictable and somewhat conservative. Here's how I might modify the outfit to better align with my style personality:

- change out the conservative white shirt to a *creative* graphic tee

- change out the predictable black jeans to *modern* black leather culottes

- change out the timeless cream bag to a *modern* red one

- keep the same blazer and same loafers.

Now my outfit aligns with my style personality. It is *tailored, polished, modern* and *creative*, instead of *conservative, predictable* and *timeless*. By identifying – and verbalising – the words that describe an outfit or particular item that doesn't quite feel like 'you', you can start to make the necessary tweaks in a much more informed way. When you know how to make your outfits align with your style personality, you will also be able to make more objective decisions when you go shopping.

And remember, only *you* know if something feels right or wrong. No one can tell you how you feel in an outfit. The most stylish items that look amazing on someone else might feel completely wrong on you. But when you know your style personality, you will have a foolproof strategy to ensure you feel your best in your clothes every day. Let's look at one more example.

Only *you* know if something feels right or wrong.

Leah's style personality

Leah works part-time as a creative arts teacher in an inner-city school. She lives with her partner and two children and has a holiday house on the coast about a two-hour drive from home. Leah splits her time between her home in the suburbs and her new holiday house on the coast. At home, she enjoys going on bike rides, cooking and watching her children play sport, and every alternate weekend she's renovating the holiday house, walking along the beach or reading a book.

Leah looked through her wardrobe to identify key items and created three outfits across different activities that she wears them for.

- Going to work: *colourful, relaxed, playful, approachable.*

- Watching children play sport: *relaxed, quirky, colourful, playful.*

- Weekend at the holiday house: *relaxed, approachable, fun.*

Reviewing these three outfits reveals a clear theme of colour and pattern and no black. Her looks include lots of baggy pants and colourful shoes including sneakers. All Leah's outfits are relaxed on the body – nothing is tight or fitted and there is no sign of anything tailored, classic or corporate. In summary, there's a *relaxed* energy and a considered use of colour and pattern to portray someone who is *fun* and *playful,* who feels *approachable* and is not too serious.

Leah's style personality: *relaxed, fun, playful, approachable.*

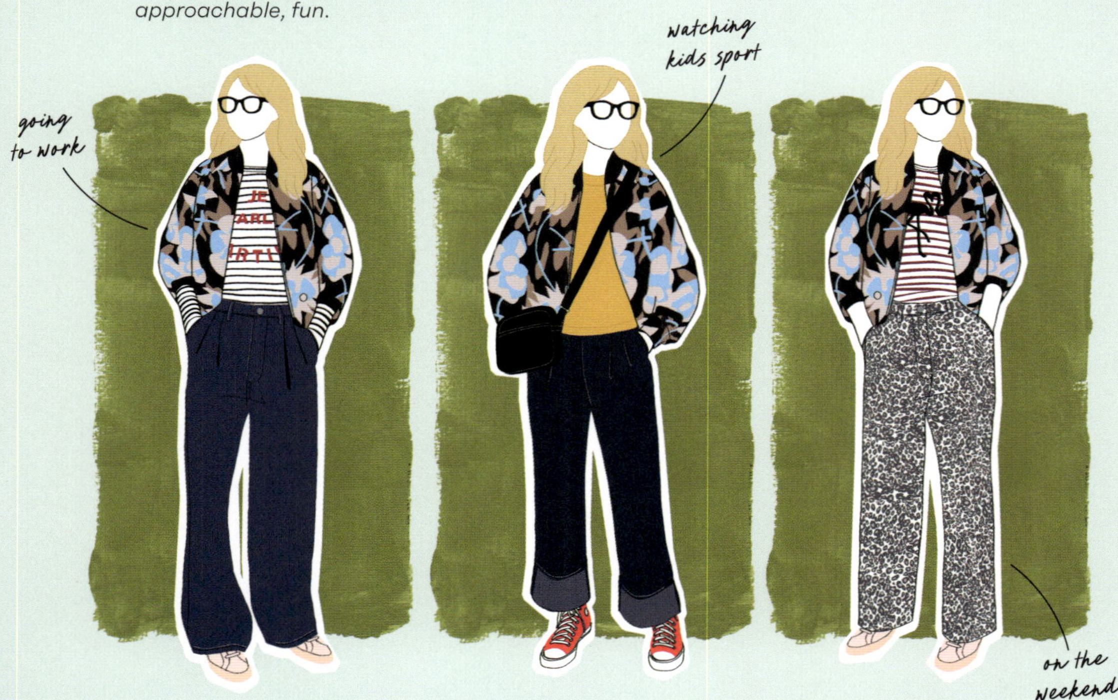

Style to suit the occasion

There are always certain occasions and situations that require us to adhere to a dress code or a set of standards. In these circumstances, while we might need to compromise, we can still portray our style personalities. Let's look at a few examples.

The funeral: Asha

Asha's style personality: *sexy*, *feminine*, *bold*, *colourful*.

Asha feels her best in feminine dresses and bright colours and loves to accentuate her waist and show off her toned, shapely legs, so on most days you'll find her in a mid-thigh dress or skirt with a belted waist. She's also quite fond of a high heel and is very rarely seen in flat shoes.

A typical outfit for Asha is a pink peplum jacket, a pussybow blouse tucked into a thigh-length pink pencil skirt with pointed-toe heels, a pop of red lipstick and a ladylike handbag.

To tweak her outfit for a funeral, Asha wears her classic navy jacket and a knee-length navy pencil skirt. She still chooses her favourite pointed-toe *bold* red stilletos and *feminine* pussybow blouse but instead of leaving the neckline open, she ties it up. Asha also maintains her signature red lip, which is always *colourful* and *sexy*. In this way, she respects the solemn occasion but still wears an outfit that aligns with her style personality.

The job interview: Cindy

Cindy's style personality: *eclectic*, *bohemian*, *quirky*, *relaxed*.

Cindy knows first impressions count, and while her natural instinct is to throw on something very casual, boho and super comfortable, she needs to present a more polished image for a job interview. She also needs to 'do' her hair and wear just a touch of make-up.

A typical outfit for Cindy is a midi-length tiered floral dress, a vintage leather jacket and biker boots with her natural wavy hair worn out and untamed.

To adjust her look for the interview, Cindy wears one of her favourite *bohemian* style dresses and works it back with a second-hand pinstripe blazer that adds some polish to the outfit, while also creating an *eclectic* pattern clash. She rolls up the sleeves to feel less corporate. She wears her hair slicked back in a low ponytail and adds some statement glasses and a pop of lipstick. She chooses to polish up some comfortable old loafers and adds a cute pair of patterned ankle socks. Cindy feels polished enough for the occasion but also feels like herself: *relaxed* and a bit fun and *quirky*.

The presentation awards: Marika

Marika's style personality: *sporty, casual, active, androgynous.*

Marika is a high school physical education teacher and spends most of her weekends playing or coaching sport, so activewear and team uniforms are on high rotation. It's the annual awards night for her basketball club and the dress code stipulates 'smart-casual'.

A typical outfit for Marika is baggy jeans, a hoodie and sneakers.

To dress for the awards but still express her style personality, Marika chooses her 'best' sneakers and gives them a buff and polish. She borrows a friend's suit – a modern, oversized blazer and tailored pants – and wears it with her favourite sports jersey with the club's name and logo emblazoned on the chest. Along with a slicked-back bun and a dash of mascara, she feels comfortable: *casual* but smart, elevated but relaxed, *sporty* but with some edge, able to move around and be *active* – balancing her own personality with the event's dress code.

A few words with a lot of power

The words you have selected for your style personality carry a lot of weight and can really help fine-tune your outfit decisions. Keep them somewhere you can easily see them when getting dressed; for example, I have mine printed in large text on the back of my wardrobe door. Remember to look at them when shopping too. My tip is to save them somewhere on your phone – you could even save them under 'Style Personality' in your contacts.

Soon these words will be top of mind, every day, when getting dressed. You'll start to ask yourself, 'Do I look x, y, z?' And if not, you'll have the tools to adapt. Just like that.

When you stay true to your style personality with every outfit you choose, it is possible to feel your true self in every situation. By doing these activities and having these conversations with yourself, you will start to understand how clothing can truly make you feel incredible every day.

3. MASTER THE THREE CS

You now have a clear idea of your wardrobe purpose and have identified your style personality. But how do we use this knowledge to shop with greater intention and cultivate a great wardrobe that both meets our needs and expresses our personal style? One of the dangers of defining our wardrobes is feeling too restricted in our choices – it's one of the things I personally find frustrating about capsule wardrobes. So, here is my secret antidote.

Let me introduce you to the **Three Cs: core**, **charisma** and **crush** – the three principal categories of your wardrobe and the foundations of fabulous outfit building. Knowing how they work, both together and separately, will ensure that no matter what you're wearing, you'll always feel like you and never feel bored with your choices. As your style evolves, so too will the items that make up your Three Cs. These little gems will ensure you build a wardrobe with maximum functionality, wearability and individuality.

I think it's a fair assumption that most of us want to buy less and buy better – we know that overconsumption and textile waste are huge problems and their impact on the environment is catastrophic. Fashion is fast, trends are even faster and it's very easy to get caught up in the hype and cycle of new, new, new. If, like me, you want to free yourself from this relentless pressure, this magical trio will help you be a more mindful and successful shopper, no matter your budget. Using the Three Cs when shopping, you'll find it much easier to decide where (and if) a piece belongs in your wardrobe and ultimately how much money you want to spend on it.

Core

As the word suggests, your **core** wardrobe is what you wear most of the time. As such, it's a big slice of your 80 per cent 'everyday' wardrobe. These pieces offer you the most versatility, wearability and functionality, and they tend to have the longest lifespan. Items you have multiples of are likely to be part of your core wardrobe. They are the pieces you're often drawn to when you walk into a store or are shopping online; the ones that align most strongly with the three primary words you identified as your style personality and that best fit your wardrobe purpose.

My core wardrobe is mostly blazers and jeans. I own many variations in different cuts, colours, fabrics, textures, shapes and sizes but, essentially, they're all blazers and jeans. They're my go-to when I want to feel like me. They're the pieces I often choose to invest in because I know they'll get worn a lot. Your core pieces might be beautifully patterned dresses that you wear all throughout the year, with sandals and sunnies in summer and with tights, boots and a turtleneck in winter. Or perhaps your core pieces are statement sneakers in all sorts of brands, colours and styles. Whatever they are, these non-negotiable, feel-good items are what make you feel unequivocally you.

For all these reasons, they are also likely to be the pieces that you invest the most in – whatever that looks like to you and your unique budget. For some, an investment piece might be $100, for others it might be $2000. Relative to your overall budget, these items cost the most. And yet, over their lifetime, they may well be the cheapest to own. If they are good quality and comfortably fit your core wardrobe, you are likely to wear them on high repeat, which brings their cost-per-wear right down. Understanding how this equation works, which I explain in detail back on page 20, is why you can be more comfortable investing in these items.

Charisma

Charisma pieces are an extension of your core items but with a little more personality, variation or points of difference. Your charisma pieces probably align with one or two of your style personality words but not all of them. This is because your wardrobe's charisma pieces are what set you apart from someone else with a similar style personality. They are the part of your wardrobe that makes you feel unique, and the reason why, even in a room full of people adhering to a dress code, no one is dressed exactly the same.

My charisma pieces include jeans but not as you know them. They might have an unusual silhouette such as the barrel-leg, a fringed hem, an exaggerated cuff or a statement rear pocket. I can mix my charisma pieces with my core when I want to elevate or change things up with a little something unexpected. I don't need a lot of charisma in my wardrobe but I do think it's important to have a few pieces, as should you.

If you're a sneaker devotee, you might have your core range of classic, white sneakers and then a selection of options with charisma, such as a pair of gold sneakers you wear when you need to feel a bit glam, chunky high-tops for when you're hanging out at weekend kids sport and one designer pair so outrageously over the top that every time you wear them people notice!

It's important that your charisma pieces still align with your core because these are what you'll be wearing most of the time. The ratio of core to charisma pieces in your wardrobe is completely up to you. One person's charisma wardrobe will look different from the next because what is considered unique or unusual will be subjective from one person to the next. They are determined by our style personality and whether we like to take risks or play it safe when it comes to getting dressed.

The difference between core and charisma

Core and charisma pieces are the workhorses of your wardrobe, fitting neatly into your 80 per cent wardrobe purpose, and both firmly expressing the defining aspects of your style personality. So how can you tell them apart? Let's use Indi and Steph as an example.

Indi and Steph are friends. As professional women in their thirties, with no children and active social lives, their wardrobe purposes are similar. So too are their style personalities, which they describe as *modern*, *minimalist* and *classic*. Their core pieces are mostly relaxed contemporary suiting separates, wide-leg pants, simple tops and tanks in block colours, jeans in classic colours and trench coats.

One Saturday they walk into one of their favourite boutiques, immediately and instinctively separating, one going left, one going right – they know what they like and don't rely on each other to make decisions. They meet at the fitting rooms, each with a few garments folded over their arms, and briefly show each other what they've chosen, then start trying on their pieces.

Indi comes out first, wearing a beautifully tailored navy blazer with a matching pair of full-length, wide-leg trousers that fall neatly to her ankle. She is wearing her loafers and loves the way the trousers complement them. She can also see how the navy blazer will work with all her jeans, other suit pants she owns and some of her work dresses. She thinks about how she can wear the pants in summer with sandals and a tank, perhaps with her classic camel trench.

In choosing the set, Indi has leant more heavily into the minimalist and classic components of her style personality. For her, the suit will fit within her *core* wardrobe, getting lots of wear and offering good value for money over time.

Steph, on the other hand, emerges in a stunning rust-coloured blazer and matching trousers. The blazer has an exaggerated shoulder and she has deliberately sized up for a relaxed look. The trousers have front pleats and sit fashionably cropped on the leg.

Steph loves the colour: it feels so fresh to her and like nothing else in her wardrobe. She envisages how it will complement and modernise all the classic colours in her wardrobe. The blazer has enough room that she can wear it in winter over a chunky rollneck jumper, and she loves how she can effortlessly push up the sleeves to make it feel more casual. The trousers are classic and tailored enough to be able to wear to the office but not so dressy that she can't imagine wearing them on weekends with a t-shirt and sneakers.

In selecting the rust-coloured suit, Steph has leant more heavily into the modern aspect of her style personality and chosen a colour outside her core set. For her, these pieces extend her core wardrobe in a fresh way but still lean into its principles and work back with all her clothes for all occasions ensuring they will get a lot of use. For Steph, this is a *charisma* purchase.

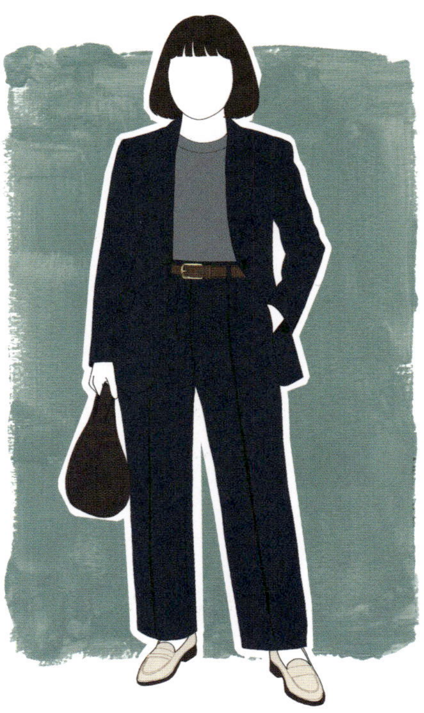

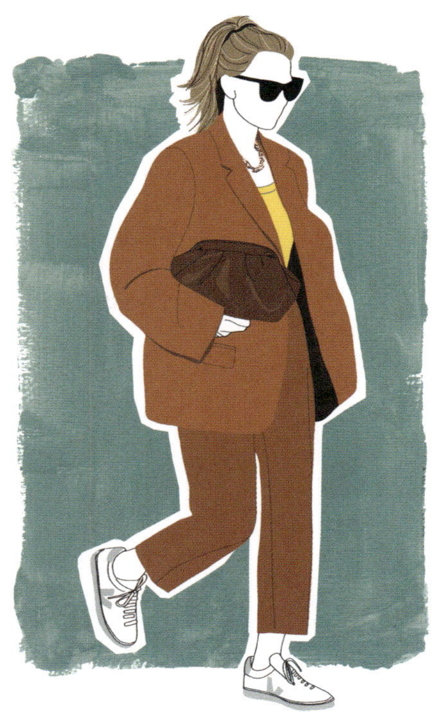

Crush

You know when you see something new, perhaps a new trend that keeps popping up on social media, and you think to yourself, 'Ooh, I love that!' Well, those are our **crush** pieces. They're the things we don't really 'need' but they elicit a sense of urgency or intrigue, a fleeting passion that makes our hearts flutter, even though we know it likely won't last forever.

Your crush portion of your wardrobe should be the feel-good pieces that you introduce periodically to have some fun with, to experiment with and to inject some freshness into your outfits. They might be those pieces that you 'had to have' at the time but when you look back, you think, 'What was I thinking?' And that's completely normal and okay, as long as you feel amazing while you're wearing them and you find a good home for them once you're ready to let them go (i.e. donate, resell, repurpose).

When considering a crush piece we should ask ourselves, 'Will I feel more current if I add this to my wardrobe?' or 'I do love this now but am I going to wear it next year?' If you know it's going to be a fairly short-term fling, this is a surefire sign it's a crush item. These pieces should take up minimal space in our wardrobes, because when our wardrobes are full of crush items, we're more likely to have a 'nothing to wear' moment as there are no core items to bring our outfit together. Or perhaps when we do get dressed top to toe in our crush pieces, we feel like we're wearing a costume. Something is just not right. We don't feel like ourselves.

A crush should work with your core and charisma pieces. Always. After all, you still want the overall look to feel like you, even as you experiment with new colours, silhouettes, patterns or textures. They might be a modern version of what you already have, such as a studded loafer, or be completely different from anything else you have, such as a feather-trimmed sequin skirt, but they should always be something you just *love*. A crush should *never* make us feel guilty; they're an integral part of the modern wardrobe. Without the addition of a crush every now and then, our clothes can feel a bit static. I think it's okay to buy something inexpensive that you feel fabulous in, wear it to death for a season, then let it go when it no longer brings you joy.

For this reason, our crush pieces are more likely to be less expensive; they're fun but they're not worth the kind of investment you'd make on something that feels more aligned with your core.

Story of a crush

The humble ballet flat became 'cool' again in 2023 and, as with any resurgence of a wardrobe classic, it evolved, this time producing the mesh ballet flat. Designed to subtly reveal toes and pedicures, it was certainly a style that turned heads and divided opinions, especially the pairs embellished with crystals.

I had already embraced the return of the ballet flat (more easily than I would ever have predicted given how I wore them to death in the early 2000s) so the idea of a mesh version was something to consider. Did they intrigue me? Yes. Did I think they were interesting but fleeting? Yes. Did I develop a bit of a crush on them? *Yes.*

The catalyst for deciding to add this crush to my wardrobe was thanks to a client. Let's just say I had mesh shoe envy! Jeni turned up to our meeting wearing a nude version of a very popular mesh ballet flat and they looked great! They added interesting texture, a point of difference and a modern update to her simple, stylish outfit. I was convinced. But did I want to spend a lot of money on them? No.

So, I didn't. I added a pair of mesh ballet flats to my wardrobe that season – embellished and all! – and they became part of my rotation of elevated flats that I wore with my core wardrobe of blazers, suits and jeans. I didn't spend a lot of money on them (even though I was coveting a very expensive pair) but they added a fun, new dimension to my outfits, just like they did for Jeni, and when I wore them, I felt cool and modern.

By the end of spring/summer 2025, you could literally buy a version of them from every high-street brand. It was at this point that the style lost its appeal for me. They'd served me well, and I wore them enough to justify the cost-per-wear. Later that year I decided I no longer liked them and donated them to my local op shop. But for as long as my crush lasted, it was super fun! Looking at these two images on the next page you can see how I used my crush piece – the embellished ballet flat – to update my core and charisma-based outfits.

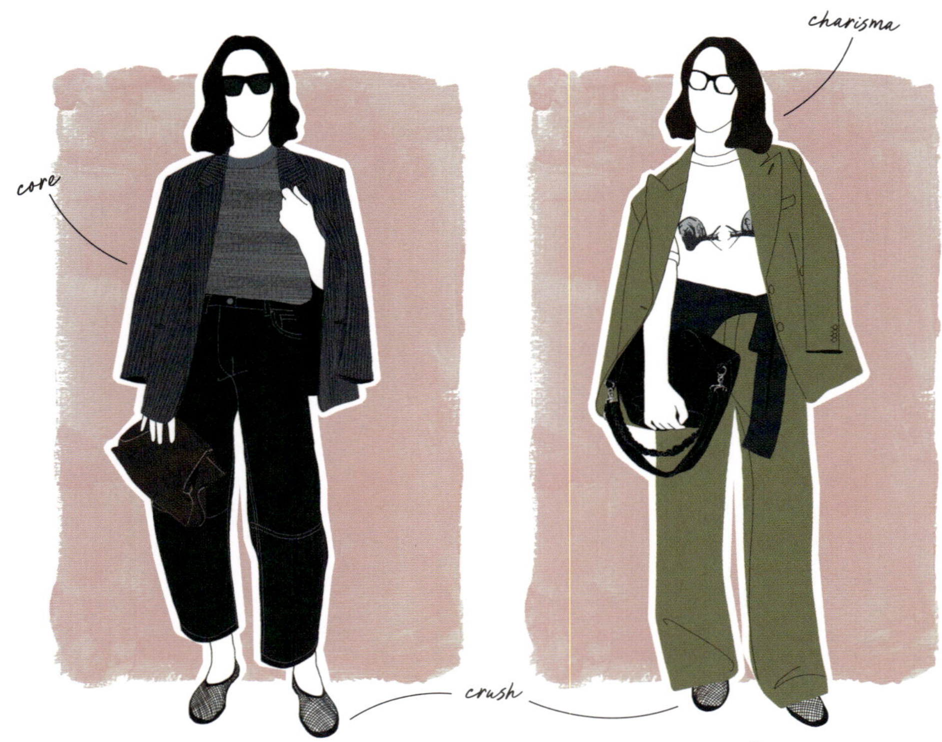

How to use the Three Cs to be a better shopper

Using your Three Cs while shopping can really help with decision-making: whether it's worth it, whether you'll wear it and, ultimately, whether you need it. When you're considering if you should add something new to your wardrobe, your first question should be, 'Which of the Three Cs would this be: core, charisma or crush?' Think of them like this:

Core – your wardrobe's heart.

Charisma – your wardrobe's personality.

Crush – your wardrobe's fun.

Apart from how they work to serve your wardrobe purpose, this approach should also help with your purchasing decisions. Core pieces are integral to your style personality and will get major use in your wardrobe over many years, so you can afford to spend more on them. Charisma pieces are slightly riskier, being a fresh colour or an updated silhouette, but will certainly get good use and are something you can spend well on. Crush items on the other hand are deliberately trend driven and a bit of fun, so not something you want to spend too much on.

Wendy, a corporate lawyer

Wendy has a senior role in a big, conservative law firm. It involves long hours, and a lot of client engagement and public speaking. Her style is conservative and classic, and she feels most herself in well-cut blazers and trousers in navy, black or cream. On her days off, she lives in jeans, t-shirts and sneakers.

Wardrobe purpose: corporate office, public speaking events, client events.

Style personality: *classic, conservative, polished, corporate, feminine.*

Shopping for Wendy's core wardrobe is always pretty straightforward. Every couple of years she replaces a well-worn navy suit with a new, slightly more modern one. For example, the blazer might be slightly longer or the trousers might have a slightly wider leg. She is always happy to invest in these pieces because she knows she'll wear them on high rotation.

While her suiting is on the *conservative* side, Wendy likes to add *feminine* touches with her blouses, skirts and shoes. She adds some charisma to her wardrobe by choosing a *feminine* cream silk shirt with a statement pussybow, a *classic* black pencil skirt with an embossed lace overlay and some leopard-print slingbacks.

During a recent shopping trip, Wendy spots a couple of crush pieces: a fun pair of embellished white sneakers and a 'cool' pair of jeans. Adding these helps Wendy avoid feeling 'too conservative' by adding a playful and modern touch to her *classic* wardrobe. She knows she'll wear the sneakers both on the commute to work and on the weekend. Her new 'mum' jeans update her skinnies, which her kids have been telling her to get rid of for years!

Core: tailored separates, blazers, cropped pants, shirt dresses, kitten heels, coats.

Charisma: pussybow silk blouses, lace pencil skirt, leopard-print heels, crushed velvet navy blazer.

Crush: embellished sneakers, mum jeans.

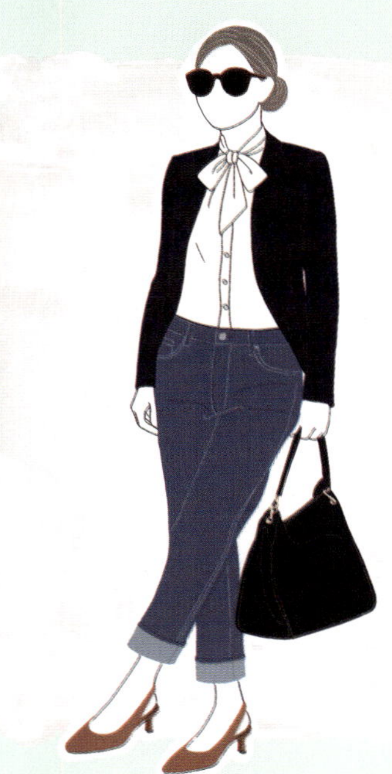

Adina, an apprentice hairdresser

Adina is a hairdresser who loves the live music scene. She has a strong sense of personal style and only wears black. She has a defined look with a rock 'n' roll edge, and she buys a lot of her clothes second-hand and from vintage stores.

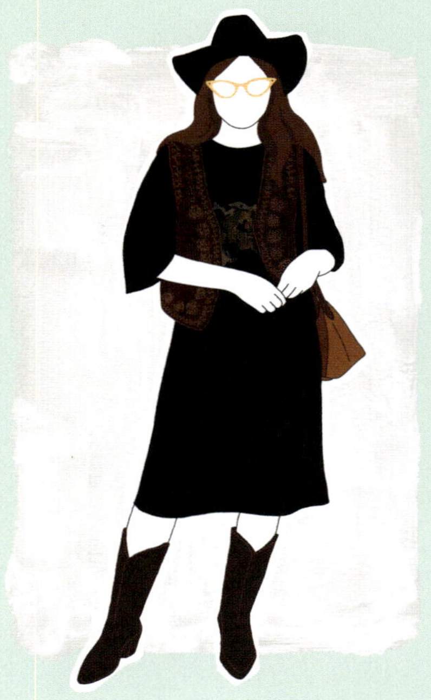

Wardrobe purpose: part-time hairdresser, part-time bartender, live music gigs.

Style personality: *rock 'n' roll, edgy, monochromatic, vintage.*

Adina's core wardrobe is made up of black skinny jeans, combat boots, vintage band t-shirts, leather jackets and slip skirts. You could describe this as her 'signature style'. When Adina scours her local second-hand and *vintage* stores, she looks for her charisma items because she knows this is where she can find pieces that are more likely to be one-offs and unique.

Sticking with her *monochromatic* scheme, she spots a fabulous pair of black cowboy boots with cool contrast stitching, which will be a great alternative to her usual combat boots. She can mix up her *rock 'n' roll* look by wearing them with her black skinnies or her slip skirts for live music gigs. Adina then spots a cool pair of vintage glasses – a classic crush piece. She doesn't need reading glasses but she loves how they add a retro vibe to her look. She thinks she might try these on her hairdressing days, along with her band t-shirts and black jeans.

Core: black skinny jeans, black combat boots, vintage band t-shirts, black slip skirts.

Charisma: cowboy boots, men's waistcoats, lace dresses, men's oversized vintage blazer.

Crush: vintage cowboy hat, vintage glasses.

Feelings and the Three Cs

Never underestimate your feelings when it comes to your personal style. They are so instrumental that they will have their own chapter later in the book! Focusing on and tuning in to how something makes you feel is an important strategy when buying something new and deciding where it fits into the Three Cs.

When considering core items, we should have a strong attraction to these pieces that allows us to visualise how they will work with the rest of our wardrobe. When we are attuned to these feelings the value of the items becomes more obvious. We know they're a good buy.

When we think of adding charisma pieces to our wardrobe, a different thought process comes into play. We want these pieces to be a little bit different, slightly special, unique. What feelings do they elicit in you? For example, for my own wardrobe, I identified barrel-leg jeans as an item with charisma, providing me with a feeling of being modern, unique and daring. For you, the same style might provoke a feeling of coolness, edge or youth. There's no right or wrong, it's just how we feel!

You may have already noticed that there can be a fine line between charisma and crush items and, ultimately, it's about how long you envision wanting to wear a piece for. A crush can give us a feeling of excitement, joy and happiness but it might be worth asking yourself if it will provoke those same feelings in six weeks, six months or twelve months. The longer you're likely to wear it, the more money you can consider investing. If a potential new purchase is only a short-term fling (which is fine!), then as a crush you'll want to spend less.

Now that I've introduced you to the Three Cs, you're going to feel more in charge of your personal style, feel more in tune with your shopping habits, and be better able to articulate what your wardrobe does and doesn't need. Whether your wardrobe spans three rooms in your house or one rack, the principles of the Three Cs are the same. If you keep these top of mind when shopping, you'll find yourself with a wardrobe that always feels aligned to your style and you'll always have something great to wear, whether reaching for a tried-and-true core piece, a charisma piece with a little more personality or a new crush you're flirting with.

The black pant,
as we know it today,
has been
declassified.

4. DECLASSIFY YOUR WARDROBE

Have you ever bought a pair of black tailored pants and only ever worn them to work or occasionally on a weekend with a nice blouse and heels to go out for dinner?

When I started styling, back in 2007, it was common for me to help clients find a fabulous pair of black pants for the office or nights out. Every woman had a pair of black pants that she kept for such occasions, because 'everyone needed a black pant in their wardrobe' . . . didn't they? And at the time, I would agree: 'Yes, you do.' But this item had little function outside of those two purposes.

Over the years, I've seen the classic black pant evolve, not only in its style but also in its purpose and functionality. The black pant, as we know it today, has been **declassified**. And if yours haven't by now, then they sure will be after you've read this chapter!

Traditionally, many items of clothing have been purchased to suit a particular need or occasion. The point of declassifying our wardrobes, however, is to wear our clothes in multiple ways and for multiple purposes. The result? An endless, hardworking, multifunctional wardrobe. Clothes no longer need to be pigeonholed into acting only for a certain purpose – they can be worn however and wherever we want to. That's not only exciting but also good news for our budgets.

This chapter is all about looking at our wardrobes with fresh eyes, getting more value out of our pieces and thinking outside the box when it comes to wearing and styling our clothes. First, let's look at the classic items that have been traditionally worn only for specific purposes, and I'll show you how you might wear them a little differently.

The black pant

Let's style this hard-working piece with other items in your wardrobe to show you how you might wear them – yes, to the office or a dressy dinner, but in other ways too.

The classicist: styles her black pants with a classic white shirt. She ties a black-and-white striped knit over her shoulders. To introduce a touch of contrast, she adds a camel trench coat as her top layer, wears a pair of two-tone ballet flats and carries a tan handbag.

The modern minimalist: wears her black pants with a white t-shirt and beige blazer. She styles this with black loafers and a black handbag.

The on-the-run mum: keeps this fun and comfortable by wearing her black pants with a white tee, a floral bomber jacket and bright green sneakers. Her crossbody bag adds a stylish and practical accessory.

↘ **The creative:** cuffs her black pants to show off her cute yellow socks and brown loafers. She wears a vintage blue denim jacket with a white shirt, a striped men's tie and red statement reading glasses.

The corporate: wears a cream silk shirt and black tailored jacket to match her black pants, accessorising these with black heels, a black belt and a black tote bag.

The possibilities don't end there but as you can see, the black pant has functionality well beyond a single use.

Notice that I'm not specifying the style or type of black pant? Yours might be cropped and mid-rise with a cigarette leg in 100 per cent wool. Someone else's might be a high-rise, full-length, elasticised waist, wide leg in a soft drapey viscose. Mine might be a super-high rise with exaggerated front pleats, a curved leg and a wide cuff in a stiff drill cotton. While the style of our black pants will differ, the variety of ways we can style them is endless once we declassify them.

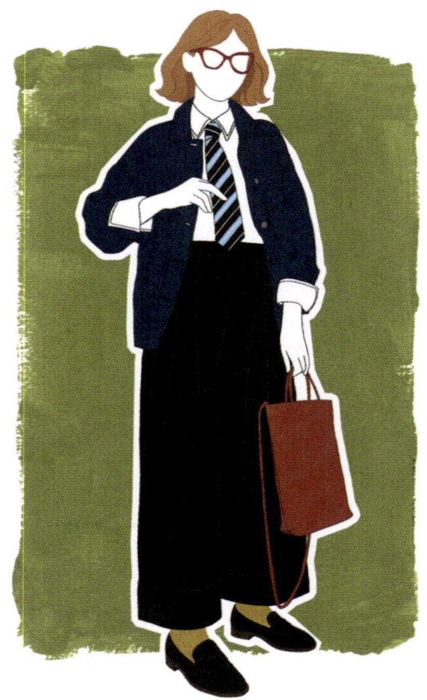

The white shirt

How many times have you read that a white shirt is a 'must have' in every woman's wardrobe? Too many to count, I'm sure! A white cotton shirt has been classified as a classic wardrobe staple; one that is fundamental to a functioning wardrobe, worn with other wardrobe staples like jeans, jackets and tailored trousers for a chic, timeless look. But what if your personal style goals are not to look classic, timeless or chic? Understanding your unique style personality can allow you to wear a white shirt in a way that feels more like you.

Whether the classic white shirt (100-per-cent cotton, button-down, pointed collar, tailored through the body) serves your personal style depends on many factors. For some this classic cut would be too stuffy and uncomfortable, others would find it annoying because it requires ironing, and others don't see it resonating with their style personality. But that doesn't mean you should discard a white shirt from your wardrobe entirely. Let me show you how a 'classic white shirt' can look very different from one wardrobe to the next.

The classicist: wears her white shirt neatly tucked into black jeans, with black ballet flats, a camel trench, a cream knit over her shoulders and a tan handbag.

The modern minimalist: has her white shirt buttoned all the way up and tucked into black pants. She adds a black blazer, black loafers and classic handbag to finish the look.

The on-the-run mum: wears her white shirt untucked over slim jeans, poking out from under a logo windcheater. She keeps the look casual with sneakers and a crossbody bag.

The creative: pops the collar on her white shirt and leaves it half untucked under a faux leather jacket. She brings out the cuffs and folds them over her jacket sleeves. She adds a vintage brooch, patterned trousers and gold ankle boots for further flair.

The corporate: tucks her white shirt into a midi pencil skirt, adds a slim belt, pointed pumps with pantihose and throws on her long black trench.

The black blazer

Hasn't the blazer come a long way? I'm not sure I even owned one until my late thirties, perhaps even my forties. As a former primary schoolteacher, I didn't need one (way too impractical). As a single woman in her early thirties, I still didn't need one (way too stuffy). And even when I started my styling business, I didn't own one as they felt way too serious for a stylist!

Those days are long gone. Now, a blazer is probably something we all own, in some form or another. It might be classic black or patterned, cropped or long, relaxed or fitted, single-breasted, double-breasted . . . the style is irrelevant. The purpose and styling options, however, are endless.

I've added a blazer of some description to the wardrobes of thousands of women, and while each of these women had a different wardrobe purpose, different style personality and different body, the blazer itself served the same function: to add polish, structure and modernity to their wardrobes. The day-to-day functionality of the blazer, and therefore its style, came down to the individual needs of the client, as you can see from the examples below.

The classicist: wears her black blazer over a striped black-and-white tee. She wears blue jeans and her classic two-tone ballet flats, and finishes the look with a black handbag.

The modern minimalist: pairs her black pencil skirt with a white-trimmed oversized black blazer, beneath which she wears a black turtleneck. Black loafers finish the look.

The on-the-run mum: wears her black blazer in a relaxed silhouette with its sleeves rolled up. Beneath it she wears a white t-shirt under blue denim overalls paired with sporty sneakers.

The creative: wears a black double-breasted blazer together with a white sheer skirt over black leggings, statement black glasses, chunky platform loafers and statement clutch.

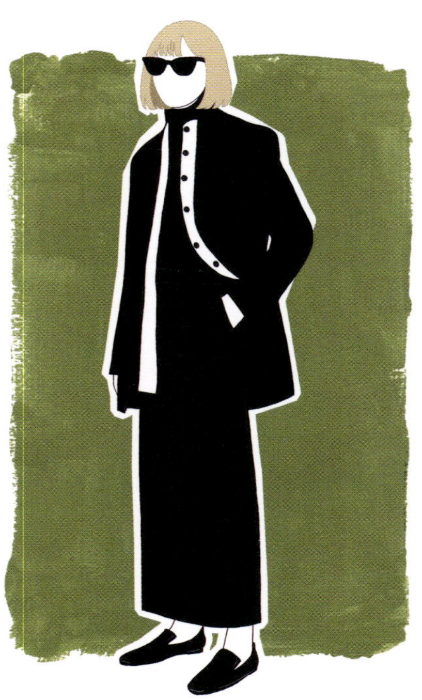

The corporate: wears her black tailored blazer with black pants, an emerald green silk blouse, black pumps and a black work bag.

Not only has your blazer become declassified in the sense that you can wear it almost anywhere (maybe even to the gym?), but 'the blazer' itself has become declassified over time because now we can buy so many variations of it, to suit our unique needs. We've never had so much choice (and so much access) to fashion from all around the world. So, if we consider the blazer in all of this, and its evolution from corporate jacket to an integral part of most wardrobes, it's quite remarkable!

How a declassified wardrobe might look

So how do you declassify your wardrobe? I'd been working with Alison for a few years, helping her build a corporate wardrobe of great suits, silk blouses and classic heels for the office. This was generally the focus of our sessions as she was very active on the weekends – playing a lot of sports, training and relaxing – so mostly wore activewear when not at the office.

After the pandemic, as with many workplaces, Alison's office took the 'dress for your day' approach to their dress code, meaning Alison now felt too 'dressed up' in her corporate suits most days. It was time to declassify her work wardrobe.

I visited her home to assess everything we'd purchased over the years, including some beautiful made-to-measure suits in classic corporate colours: black, grey and navy. Her suiting was in great condition and was still modern and relevant in terms of cut and form, and she certainly didn't want it to collect dust in her wardrobe – and neither did I. We came up with our plan of attack.

My first suggestion was to switch out her corporate heels for something more casual. Easy!

Next, we needed to split the suits into separates and looked at how we might style them with the more casual items already in her wardrobe, and those we planned to purchase, which included:

- fresh white trainers and red loafers to dress down her suits

- some classic blue jeans to wear with her suit jackets

- a couple of midi-skirts – one a pleat and one a pencil style – to feminise her suit jackets

- some simple crewneck knits for under her suits instead of silk shirts

- good quality crewneck t-shirts to simplify and modernise her suiting: a white, a graphic tee and a stripe

- a more relaxed, casual blazer in a colour different from her suits

- some non-blazer outerwear options: a modern trench and a bomber jacket.

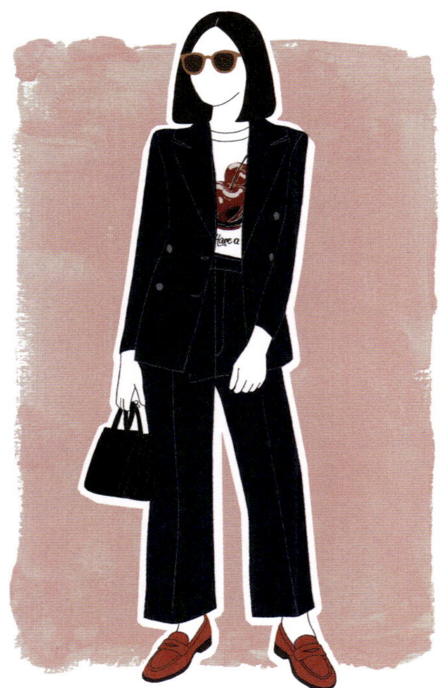

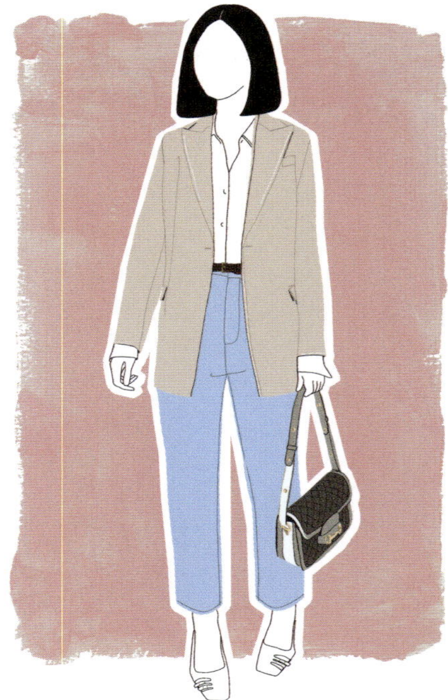

Alison could still pull out the tailored suits with her pumps and silk pussybow blouses for an important client meeting, or team that same blouse and suit jacket with jeans and a nice flat and still feel professional. She could wear a t-shirt and her casual blazer with her suit pants and a pair of smart white sneakers. We had declassified her corporate items, meaning she could still get lots of wear from them but not look too formal on days that didn't require full corporate attire.

By declassifying your wardrobe items, you get so many more opportunities to wear your clothes and to style them in ways that properly reflect your style personality instead of looking like everyone else.

Activity: Declassify your wardrobe

Take one item from your own wardrobe that you feel you have classified as serving just one or two purposes. Using a pen and paper, write down at least five new ways to style that item. Use the examples I've shared to help you with ideas. There are no wrong or right answers!

Do this activity with as many items from your wardrobe as you like. Have fun experimenting with different combinations for different occasions. If you've got the time and energy for it, try on the combinations and take photos. Keep your photos for future reference, and especially for those days when you're feeling uninspired or don't know what to wear.

A declassified approach to shopping

When we declassify items in our wardrobes, particularly the ones we spent a lot of money on, it can bring a sense of relief because we're now giving ourselves permission to wear those pieces so much more!

When considering buying something new, think about that item's use beyond what you 'traditionally' might be buying it for. If you're buying something that will serve your wardrobe purpose 20 per cent of the time, could it also apply to your 80 per cent? It may or may not, and that's okay – not everything has to tick the declassification box! But would you, for example, consider 'elevated' trackpants? Trackpants or lounge pants can indeed just be something you wear working from home, to watch TV on a Sunday night or to lie on the couch reading. But *could* that same pair of pants, if it was made of a certain fabric, in a certain style or colour, also be worn with a trench and sneakers for other activities such as popping out to the shops, heading out to a child's sporting event or a casual coffee date with a friend?

Not *everything* has to tick the declassification box!

Joy, maternity leave

Joy is a mum on maternity leave and an avid Instagram follower. She loves fashion and, despite being home with two young children, she has promised herself she won't get into a rut of only wearing leggings and activewear. She wants to make more of an effort, because it makes her feel good.

Wardrobe purpose: casual and functional clothing that is comfortable and low maintenance, with a playful and colourful feel.

Style personality: *casual, playful, laid-back.*

Joy loves jeans but just doesn't find them comfortable for her current lifestyle and wants to find something more comfortable but still stylish. Joy notices me wearing 'elevated' trackpants, and, more importantly, wearing them all the time. She sees me wear my striped joggers with everything from a kitten heel and blazer for a day of shopping to my high-tops, trench and casual crossbody bag on the weekend.

Joy is intrigued with the idea that trackpants (otherwise known as jogger pants or sweatpants) can be elevated into the everyday modern wardrobe. She's only ever worn them to play sport, to clean the house or, on the very rare occasion, to pop to the supermarket (worn under a long puffer for disguise!). Never does she think they could be a highly functional and multipurpose item in her wardrobe.

That is until she tries it. Joy buys a nice pair of red trackpants with a navy stripe down the side. She now wears them every day instead of her uncomfortable jeans: to take the kids to the park, do pickups from daycare, meet a friend for a coffee, do the grocery shopping . . . and she feels amazing. On the weekends, when she has a rare moment to herself, she teams them with her pointed boots, relaxed cashmere knit, a coat and a nice handbag to have lunch with her parents. She feels polished – and comfortable! Months later when Joy returns to work part-time she wears her sweats with a nice knit, a blazer and pointed-toe boots. She sends me a photo saying she feels fabulous. She looks it too!

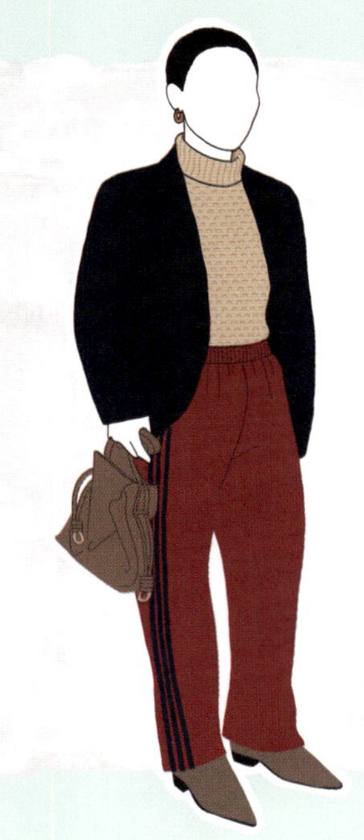

Getting more use from your 'every now and then' pieces

Let's now consider some of the less 'everyday' pieces in our wardrobes and see if we can declassify them too.

The formal dress

Would I be guessing correctly that you've got at least one 'event dress' hanging in your wardrobe, taking up space? You may have bought it for a special occasion and only worn it once, to a wedding, a formal, the races. Whatever the reason, it served its purpose, but now what?

- Without your hair and make-up done, could it work under a leather jacket, with tights and ankle boots?

- Could you wear it with sneakers, a denim jacket and a casual crossbody bag?

- Can you wear it out to dinner with flat sandals and your favourite blazer and a clutch?

Sequin anything!

There's nothing wrong with a bit of everyday sparkle, so why not try it?

- You might wear a sequin skirt with a white t-shirt, sneakers and a denim jacket.

- You could wear a sequin bomber jacket with a silky cami, jeans and flats.

- Why not try a wide-leg sequin pant with a cosy oversized knit, winter coat and boots?

Strappy summer dress

These dresses are often our go-to on summer holidays or when we want something comfortable, light and airy on our body. On other occasions, however, that same dress can feel a bit too 'summery' or exposed. But let's look at the strappy summer dress through our newly developed 'declassified' lens:

- Can you wear it over a crewneck t-shirt with a denim jacket and sandals?

- How about over a turtleneck and tights, with a blazer and ankle boots?

- And now, turned into a skirt with an oversized knit jumper, knee-high boots and an overcoat?

Summer sandals

Why let your favourite summer sandals sit in their boxes for nine months of the year when you can style them all year round? (Well, almost!)

As someone who works indoors, in either heating or air conditioning, and is on their feet a lot of the day, I have received comments on my footwear for many years. When I've posted a picture of me with bare ankles on a cold day, people say, 'Put some socks on!' or 'Aren't your ankles cold?' In contrast, when I've worn strappy heels or slingbacks with socks or tights, to indeed keep my ankles warm, I've received comments like, 'Socks and sandals, no way!' or 'You can't wear stockings with backless shoes' or 'Can you wear stockings with an open toe shoe?' My answer is usually to say, 'It mightn't be your cup of tea, but it works for me,' which it does.

By declassifying my shoe wardrobe, I get so much more wear out of my shoes and such value for money! Sure, teaming my sandals or loafers with a coloured tight or sock in winter is a fashion statement but it's also a pragmatic style choice. Wearing my ballet flats sans socks with my cropped jeans in the middle of winter for a day of personal shopping is perfectly suited to my environment (a warm – often too warm! – shopping centre) and, most importantly, my style personality. And as my personal style has become more relaxed and fluid, meaning I now wear more oversized silhouettes like wide-leg pants and jeans, I look for items that can add balance to this look. The strappy 'barely there' sandal is a great way to balance a full-length pant because it shows some skin at the foot. That's another reason that I find myself reaching for these sandals outside of summer.

- Try wearing your strappy flat sandals with a suit.

- Style strappy heels with a contrasting pair of tights, a midi-skirt and an on-trend jacket.

- Wear white strappy heeled sandals, with lurex socks, under black cropped pants, a black turtleneck and blazer.

- Wear flat strappy sandals with wide-leg jeans that fall to the floor, a simple tank and clutch.

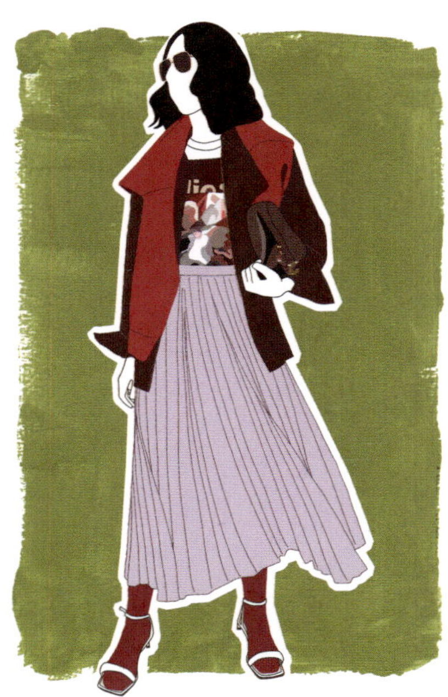

Declassified success

I've been helping clients declassify their wardrobes for years. Not only does this approach provide more styling options and outfit possibilities but ultimately it will save you money too. We've all heard the saying, 'less is more'. Well, when you declassify your wardrobe, that's exactly what you'll get! Less clothing but way more possibilities.

Have fun *experimenting* with different combinations for different occasions.

5. BUILD A MODULAR WARDROBE

I'm sure you're familiar with the 'capsule wardrobe' concept. First popularised in the 1970s by designer Donna Karan as a way to simplify one's wardrobe, reduce clutter and focus on quality over quantity, a capsule wardrobe is a curated collection of versatile clothes that can be mixed and matched to create a wide variety of outfits.

The capsule wardrobe saw a resurgence in the early 2020s, gaining widespread popularity thanks to the likes of Instagram and TikTok. As a personal stylist, I saw an exponential increase in clients coming to me with the aim of having the ultimate 'capsule'. Our social media feeds were awash with beautifully curated, minimalist outfit combinations – black pants, white shirt, blue jeans, striped t-shirt, beige trench – which looked easy, stylish and attainable. For some people, this was indeed the ultimate pain-free wardrobe; it required little thinking or imagination and was easy to pull together.

In theory, a capsule wardrobe is a great idea. Fewer clothes equal less expense, less confusion and less decision-making. But what about those of us who crave a bit more variety in our everyday style? How do we express ourselves as individuals? Well, by using the charisma and crush pieces in our wardrobes of course! Let me show you how.

The modular wardrobe

Let me introduce you to your new best friend: the **modular wardrobe**. Like the classic capsule wardrobe, this curated collection of clothes provides maximum versatility and ultimate ease but it offers more depth and variation than the classic capsule. Let's dive deeper.

The term 'modular' refers to modules, or units, that go together easily and flexibly. Think of a modular home or a modular couch. Our Three Cs are the modules of our wardrobes. Each day we reconfigure those units to create our outfit of the day (#OOTD, as tagged by content creators).

As we learnt in Chapter 3, each of the Three Cs modules is designed to perform a specific function. As the primary module, our core wardrobe contains our staple pieces that are the essence of our personal style and that we wear almost every day. When we reach for this module, we feel like ourselves. There are no restrictions as to how this module looks, what pieces are in it or how many. Mine will be different from yours because my wardrobe purpose and style personality is different from yours.

When we want to wear something that's simple and straightforward, we can create outfits using only pieces from our core module, much like a capsule wardrobe. But most of us crave more, which is why I love the Three Cs, as it gives us two more modules to play with. Our charisma module – pieces that help us differentiate our personal style from one day to the next and from other people whose core module may be very similar to our own. And our crush module, which offers even more versatility and individuality (and, I would argue, fun!) – the pieces that keep our style fresh and spark joy, for fleeting moments.

These modules can be combined, interchanged and assembled to create different outcomes. That, right there, is the true definition of a modular wardrobe. Let's look at how a modular wardrobe works in real life.

Modularity using core and charisma

My clients Vesna and Clare have very similar core wardrobes that reflect the fashion of the day. But Vesna and Clare have very different wardrobe purposes. They also have very different charisma and crush pieces.

While their common core pieces could make both women look quite similar, their charisma and crush elements allow each to express their individual style personality and wardrobe purpose.

Their common core wardrobe includes:

- tailored pants
- blue jeans
- essential white tee
- trench coat
- stylish flat shoes
- classic white sneakers
- crossbody bag.

Vesna's modular wardrobe

Vesna is semi-retired, in her sixties and a city dweller. She likes exploring new restaurants, going to the theatre and walking a lot. Her charisma and crush pieces help her express her individuality.

Charisma:

- printed silk blouses in bold colours
- high-waisted, front-pleat tailored pants in a rich burgundy
- navy velvet blazer
- white patent flats with a statement buckle
- a classic designer handbag in red.

Crush: mesh ballet flats.

Clare's modular wardrobe

Clare is in her late thirties, works full-time, has an inner-city lifestyle and lives an active single's social life.

Charisma:

- emerald green wide-leg pants
- colourful printed linen coordinated set
- red pointed-toe pumps
- gold leather clutch
- sequin butterfly brooch.

Crush: black sequin pants.

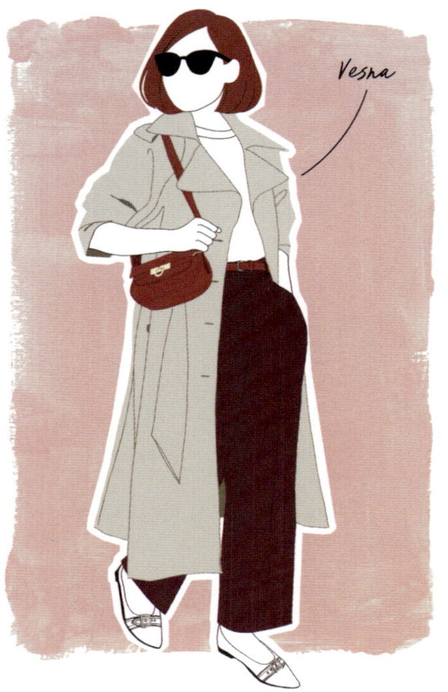

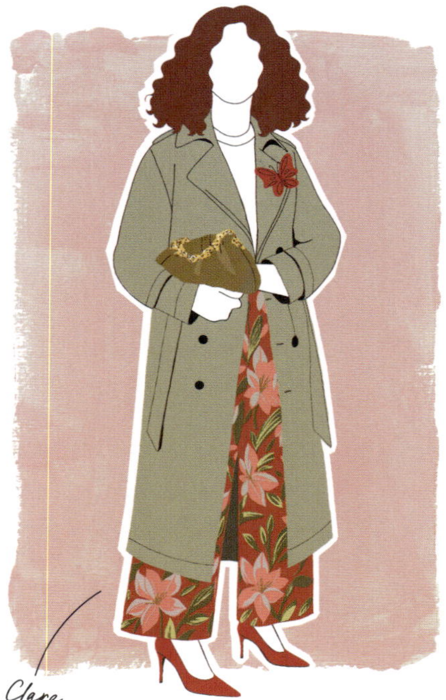

Although their core wardrobe is similar, the way Vesna and Clare style their charisma pieces with their core means they have very different looks. Adding a few crush pieces into the mix every season or so, they maintain ever-evolving wardrobes that stay fresh and interesting while still aligned with their style personalities and wardrobe purposes.

Modularity brings the difference

Without the charisma and crush modules, there's less variety, less fun and much less personality in our core wardrobes. But the beauty of combining all three is that we can have a highly curated wardrobe that is full of individuality, provides versatility and is immensely functional and, ultimately, stylish!

A modular wardrobe also allows us to build outfits using my declassification approach, taking pieces that suit one wardrobe purpose and making them work for another. Let's look at some more examples.

Anh's modular wardrobe

Anh is in her early forties. She works from home and is a mum of two. As a busy, working mum she requires a casual, functional, low-maintenance and versatile wardrobe to serve equal amounts of family time and downtime. Anh doesn't need dressy items other than for the occasional event and she prefers casual family restaurants and cafés over fancy restaurants. She prefers wash-and-wear clothing.

Core: blue jeans, black jogger pants, blue denim jacket, merino knits, striped tees, white sneakers.

Charisma: leopard-print jeans, printed puffer vest, PVC burgundy trench, colourful sneakers.

Crush: graphic tees, lurex knit top, chunky dad sandals.

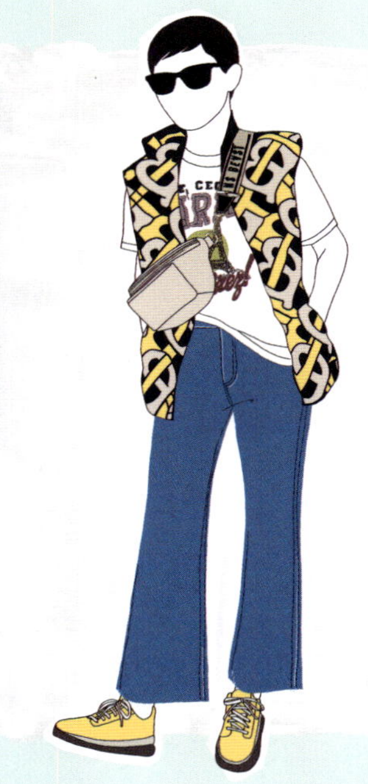

Radhika's modular wardrobe

Radhika is in her mid-twenties; a full-time social worker in a smart–casual work environment with an active social life of live music gigs and clubs. For work, Radhika's style is professional but approachable. She relies on a 'uniform' of black dresses worn all year round, seasonally adjusted by adding layers of skivvies, tights and boots for the cooler months of the year or worn with a comfortable flat or sandal and light jacket for spring and summer. Out of work, her wardrobe is a lot more 'sassy' and bold: dresses worn with heels; and she always likes to 'get dressed', even for grocery shopping. At home, she'll just wear PJs.

Core: black dresses, black long-sleeve bodysuits, black tights, black boots, black heels.

Charisma: patterned dresses, vintage silk skirts, black leather biker jacket, lurex stockings, patterned socks, leopard-print Mary Jane heels, red ankle boots.

Crush: sequin camisole, faux fur jacket.

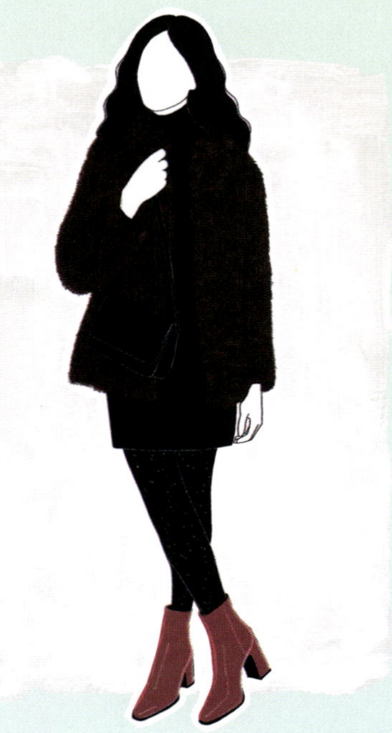

Gillian's modular wardrobe

Gillian is an inner-city lawyer in her fifties. She works full-time, with long days and not much downtime. Her professional wardrobe needs to be polished and corporate, every day. First impressions count in her line of work, and her new senior role has her working alongside some very influential people in her industry. Gillian loves to dress in a way that elicits feelings of confidence, competence and control. She has her suits and shirts made by a local tailor and invests in designer shoes and bags. When not working, Gillian enjoys quiet nights in, switching off from the world with a good book and glass of red wine, or the occasional night out with friends at a bar or fancy restaurant.

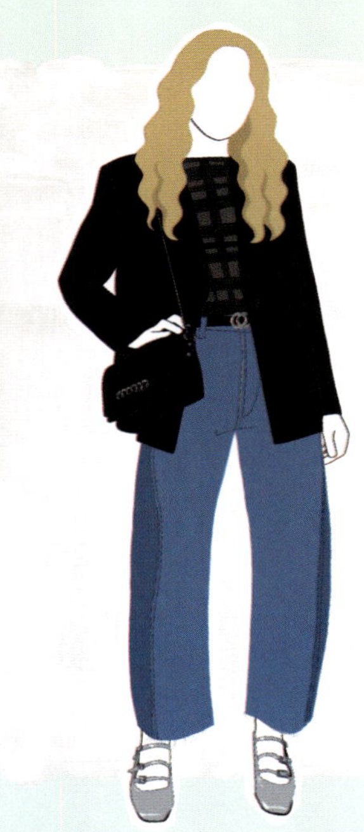

Core: black pencil skirt, black suit jacket, silk blouses in black, white and cream, charcoal overcoat, black trench, black pumps, black loafers.

Charisma: red patent pumps, lurex pleated skirt, silver flats, leopard-print loafers, checked top, designer bum bag, houndstooth blazer.

Crush: high-street mustard pants suit, multi-coloured sneakers, barrel-leg jeans.

Modularity means individuality

Each of the examples in this chapter – Vesna and Clare, as well as Anh, Radhika and Gillian – all look at their wardrobes through a multifaceted lens. They deliberately buy pieces to fulfil their core, charisma and crush modules, giving them high-functioning, variable and unique wardrobes that suit their individual wardrobe purpose. Though some share a core wardrobe, their wardrobes look quite different thanks to their charisma and crush pieces, and these also keep their style fresh and help ensure they don't tire of their core collection. As such, each of their wardrobes expresses their style personality, whether standing on the sidelines at Saturday sport, meeting a friend for a drink, hosting book club or presenting a case in court. And that is the power of the modular wardrobe.

A highly curated wardrobe is full of *individuality*, provides *versatility* and is *immensely functional* and, ultimately, *stylish*!

Two

Developing Your Style

I'm a firm believer
in *not letting* your
body shape dictate
your personal style.

6. EMBRACE YOUR SHAPE

You've now identified your wardrobe purpose, determined your style personality and learnt about the Three Cs and the modular wardrobe – an organised one at that! You're learning to look at your wardrobe with fresh eyes, to see all the possibilities sitting right in front of you. Your confidence is growing. You're making better choices when shopping, thinking more pragmatically about your spending, and caring less about fitting in or conforming to old-fashioned notions about how women should dress.

How are you feeling . . . relieved, excited, nervous? All of the above?

The chapters you've read and activities you've completed so far have prepared you for this one, which is not only central to this book but to my career.

Embrace the shape you have

I'm a firm believer in not letting your body shape dictate your personal style. What you choose to wear should be completely up to you, regardless of your body type. Shortly, I'll take you through a brief overview of how fashion has changed through the centuries and you'll see that an 'ideal body shape' is simply a myth based on current social norms – the 'perfect' body shape and fashion silhouette has changed so many times that it simply can't exist. That's why I believe so strongly in embracing the shape you have.

As someone who puts themselves out there on social media to educate women, I have received many comments about my body because I use my own body to demonstrate (as do most content creators). We come in all shapes and sizes, and, just as I advise you to do – I work with the body I have. My intention is not to force my body shape or silhouettes of choice onto anyone. I deliberately don't mention body shape, and I certainly don't mention size or age; instead, I aim to provide encouragement, guidance and inspiration driven by confidence and creativity. But I've received comments such as 'Everything looks good on you because you're slim', 'You can wear that because you're tall', 'Can you show this on a "real" woman?' and 'But how can I wear that if I'm [insert any body shape]?'

I understand where these questions are coming from. Over several generations we've been programmed to feel a need to conform to certain standards or body ideals. I know I'm tall and lean – that's just me. My mother and father were very tall, so it was natural that I would be too. I acknowledge that my height and size has benefitted me in my work with fashion brands on social media but that doesn't mean I look 'better'. Does being this shape or size automatically make me a good stylist? Absolutely not. Does it mean clothes look different on me from how they would on someone else? Yes, because no item of clothing looks the same on any two people.

As humans – and I'd argue, especially as women – we have a natural instinct to compare ourselves to others, which we do in many aspects of everyday life. We've *always* compared our looks with those around us, quite possibly ever since clothing was invented! But of course, we marvellous humans come in all shapes and sizes and we look different and feel different. Sure, this is partly due to our height, shape, complexion and hairstyle but, mostly, it's due to our individuality. The only person who sees and experiences the world the way you do is you. So, I'd like to encourage you to let your outward expression reflect who you are on the inside by finding the joy in styling and dressing to express your truest, happiest self. But first, it may help to take a quick look through just how much fashion has changed through the centuries.

The only person who *sees* and *experiences* the world the way you do is you.

A brief history of the 'ideal' body type

The era you grew up in – or are living in now – will have determined what was considered the 'ideal' body type at the time. These 'ideals' varied significantly over the past century, influenced by cultural, social, political and fashion trends. Before I talk about embracing your shape today, let's look back at the history and evolution of the female form and how what is considered 'ideal' was shaped by these factors.

1900

At the turn of the 20th century the ideal body type featured a slender, corseted waist, with a full bust and wide hips, as influenced by the Gibson Girl illustration by Charles Dana Gibson (1890). This archetype portrayed a sophisticated woman with an hourglass figure, upswept hair, high collar and elegant dress.

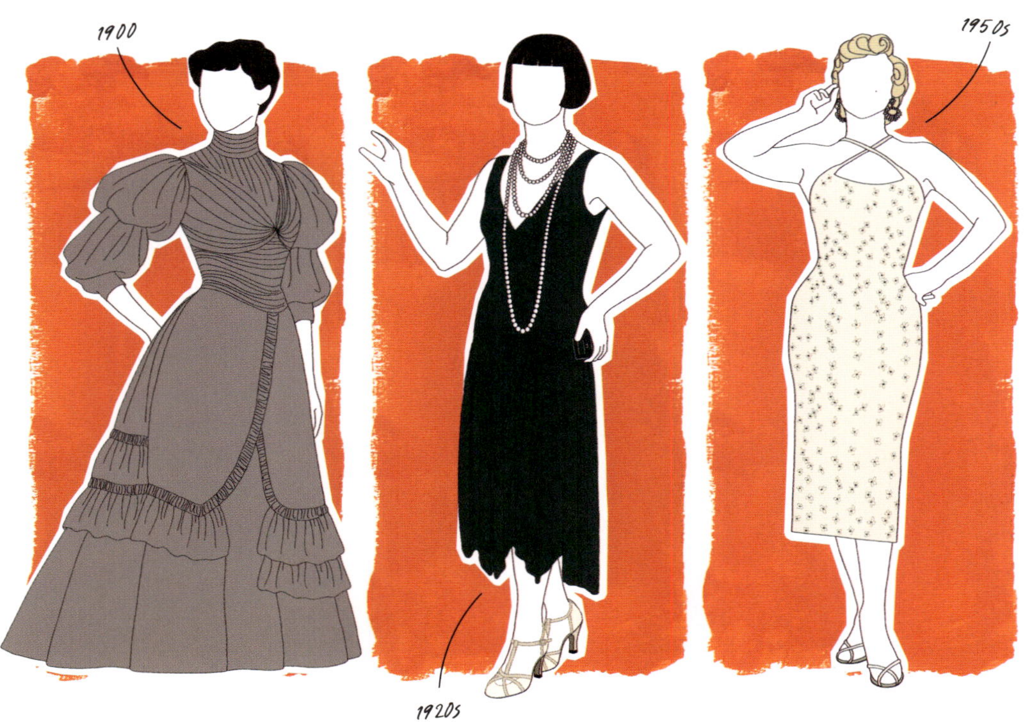

1920s

In the 1920s, the ideal shifted to a slim boyish silhouette epitomised by the flapper. Women wore shorter skirts, loose drop-waist dresses, bobbed haircuts, cloche hats and bold make-up. This style de-emphasised the bust and hips, representing modernity, freedom and changing gender roles.

1930s and 1940s

In the 1930s and 1940s, the ideal body type returned to a feminine shape with a slim waist and curves, influenced by Hollywood stars like Jean Harlow, Rita Hayworth and Lauren Bacall. Fitted bodices, flared skirts and bias-cut evening gowns in luxurious fabrics, such as satin and silk, accentuated the waist. Soft, romantic hairstyles offered elegance and escapism during the tough times of the Great Depression and World War II.

1950s

In the 1950s, the hourglass figure, embodied by Marilyn Monroe and Sophia Loren, continued to reign supreme. To enhance women's curves, fashion embraced full skirts, cinched waists and fitted bodices, while pencil skirts and jumper sets emphasised the bust and hips. This era celebrated a return to domesticity and traditional gender roles post-World War II, with fashion reflecting idealised femininity and domestic bliss.

1960s

By the 1960s, the ideal shifted again to a more slender, elongated silhouette, influenced by the mod and hippie movements. Twiggy's androgynous look, with her thin frame, short hair and large eyes, defined the decade's fashion. The mod movement embraced bold colours, geometric patterns and short hemlines, with miniskirts symbolising youthful rebellion and freedom.

The late 1960s saw the rise of the hippie movement, which favoured a more natural, less-structured look. Flowing fabrics, bell-bottoms and peasant blouses became popular, promoting a sense of individualism and countercultural values. The fashion of the 1960s was a clear departure from the formality of the 1950s, embracing a more relaxed and eclectic style.

1970s

Come the 1970s, the ideal female figure shifted to a more athletic look, popularised by icons like Farrah Fawcett and Cheryl Tiegs. Fashion embraced a casual and natural aesthetic with flowing maxi-dresses, while bell-bottom pants and peasant blouses remained popular. Farrah Fawcett's iconic poster, with her wearing a red one-piece swimsuit, showcased this era's beauty standards, while the rise of fitness culture emphasised looks that supported a healthy, active lifestyle.

1980s

In the 1980s, the ideal female body remained healthy, athletic and toned, influenced by fitness trends like aerobics and sports fashion. This era saw the rise of supermodels such as Cindy Crawford, Elle Macpherson and Naomi Campbell, who embodied this ideal. Fashion featured bold, extravagant styles with power dressing, including padded shoulders on blazers and structured suiting, reflecting women's growing professional presence. The fitness craze, led by figures like Jane Fonda, popularised brightly coloured leotards, leggings and leg warmers, reinforcing the toned, muscular body ideal.

1990s

Then, in the 1990s, the ideal body type shifted dramatically to 'heroin chic', characterised by a waifish, emaciated look with thin, pale and fragile models often sporting dark circles under their eyes. This trend, popularised by

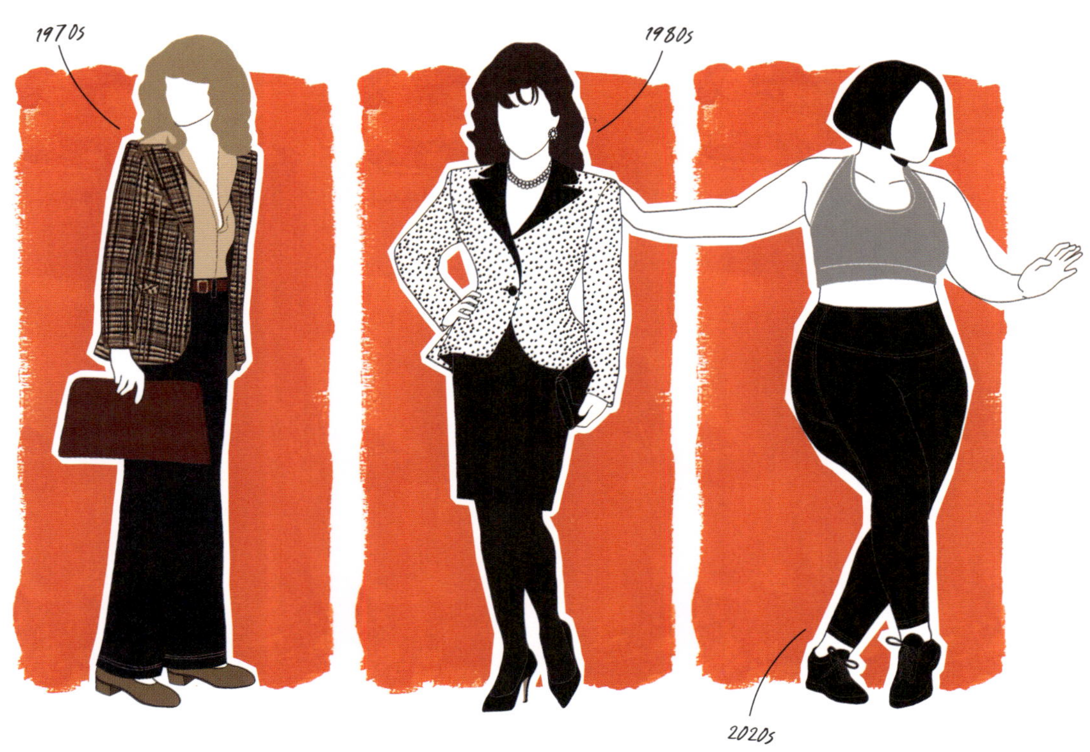

fashion figures like Kate Moss, faced significant criticism for glamorising drug use and potentially encouraging eating disorders. Fashion campaigns frequently showcased models in dishevelled, bleak settings, highlighting the grunge and underground culture of the decade and marking a stark departure from the athletic ideals of the 1980s.

2000s

The 2000s saw the continued dominance of slim figures but with increasing criticism and pushback against the unrealistic standards set by the fashion industry. Popstars like Britney Spears, Jennifer Lopez and Pink set the standard with their unapologetic expression of curves, strength and vigour. But with this came the decade of reality TV, where 'normal' people were suddenly in the spotlight, and one's weight became running commentary.

2010s

Moving into the 2010s, the rise of social media platforms like Instagram, and the body positivity movement, played crucial roles in a shift towards celebrating a wide range of body types. Brands and designers started to embrace inclusivity by featuring models of various sizes, ages, ethnicities and gender identities in their campaigns and on runways.

2020s

Today, in the 2020s, the fashion industry continues to evolve, with ongoing efforts to promote healthy, diverse and realistic body standards, along with celebrating individuality and empowering women to embrace their unique selves. However, the rise of platforms like TikTok also means that women are bombarded with images and messaging about body 'trends' more than ever.

Assets versus flaws

It's little wonder that, as women, we focus on our body shape as a pillar of our self-worth, especially when it comes to fashion and style. One minute we're supposed to be curvy and voluptuous; the next, slim and waiflike! We may fit the 'ideal' today but be out of vogue tomorrow. Think of body shape just like trends: they come, they go. There is no right or wrong, in or out, just 'preferred' standards and benchmarks that are set by extenuating factors beyond our control. It is unrealistic to try to change our bodies to match current trends – not to mention unhealthy.

I've asked clients for years, 'What do you like most about your body? What are your best bits? Your assets?' and I can guarantee that 90 per cent of women answer by telling me what they *don't* like. Why? Because many of us focus on the parts of our body we want to disguise rather than the parts we want to highlight.

Let's face it, like many things in life, when assessing our bodies we tend to focus on the negatives rather than the positives. But I'm here to encourage you to switch that thinking. When we focus on choosing clothing to 'cover up', 'hide behind' or 'disguise' part of our body, we fixate on the negative, and the process of shopping and dressing therefore becomes adverse from the outset. But when we choose clothing that 'accentuates', 'enhances', 'shows off' and 'draws the eye to' the parts of our bodies we like, feel most comfortable with and have the most confidence in, then it changes the game entirely.

Our assets don't have to be the typical body parts we might associate with body shape, like a small waist, a generous bust or balanced hips and shoulders. They can be any part of our appearance – think strong calves, thick hair, unblemished skin – and they will be determined by you, no one else.

Activity: What you like about yourself

What you need:
pen and paper

Rather than recite all the things you don't like about yourself, I want you to write down what you *do* like. What are the parts of your body that you most like to accentuate or draw attention to? What parts of your body do you want people to see? You might write down one answer to this question or many. You might struggle to write even one, but I want you to try. Here are some examples from women I've worked with who've found this task challenging:

'I really like my blue eyes.'
'I like my strong, broad shoulders.'
'I think I have a good, pert bottom.'
'I've inherited my grandmother's beautiful skin.'
'I like being tall.'

Once you've completed your list, keep it handy for the next time you're shopping or putting together an outfit from your wardrobe. Look objectively in the mirror and focus on the attributes on your list. Ask yourself, 'Does this accentuate my assets?' The answer might not always be yes, and that's okay, but the point is that you have the power to wear things or style them in a way that draws attention to the parts of your body you like most.

It can be challenging to change your mindset but just try it; one day, one outfit at a time. Trust me, when you start to think like this, the way you look at yourself will become more positive. The language you use to describe how something 'feels' will change too. You'll shop differently, you'll dress differently and you'll *feel* different.

Belle in the mirror

I first worked with Belle about a year after the birth of her first child. She had just returned to her job as a teacher two days a week, where the dress code was smart-casual. Like many new mums, Belle's shape had changed after her pregnancy, and she was feeling a bit lost with her personal style. During our initial chat, I asked, 'What do you like most about your body? What areas are you most confident drawing the eye to?'

Belle answered, 'Oh, gosh, I've never really thought about what I like about my shape! I can tell you what I don't like?'

'Let's focus on what you *do like* first,' I replied.

'Okay, that's a hard one,' she said. 'Well, I do have nice skin, slim wrists and ankles, and I do love my naturally curly hair. Does hair count?'

'Absolutely!'

Next, we looked through Belle's wardrobe and I helped her put looks together, especially for her return to work, that focused on ensuring her assets were 'on show'. I showed her how to expose her beautiful skin by pushing up the sleeves of her jackets to reveal her forearms, how to cuff her jeans and roll up the waistband of her maxi-skirts to show off her slim ankles, to open the collar of her shirts to show her decolletage and to wear her hair down to frame and highlight her face. Focusing on what Belle liked about herself instantly drew her focus away from what she didn't like, and it completely changed the way she saw herself in the mirror.

Letting go of the hypercritical self

We've all been there: standing in front of a mirror, judging and critiquing our body, assessing it from all angles. And in this moment, it doesn't take long for our hypercritical self to rear its ugly head. I've done it myself and I've been in thousands of fitting rooms and homes with other women who've done it too. Our gaze lands on the part or parts of our body we don't love. We can't look at anything else. We are fixated on our 'flaws'.

As a personal stylist, I have found this a very challenging part of my job: watching a client focus so intently on what they dislike about themselves that they can't see the big picture, that being: an outfit in its entirety. This is why acknowledging the hypercritical self and training ourselves to shift our focus from disguising our flaws to accentuating our assets is so crucial.

Referring back to your list of assets that you wrote out when looking at yourself in the mirror will help to ensure that you focus on the positives first. I'm not suggesting that this will override or counteract all negativity we might have about our bodies. But it will slowly change your mindset from being critical to being kind.

A great support in this are our friends. Think about how you often tell a friend the things you admire or like about their body. I'm sure, like me, you've said something along the lines of, 'Oh, I wish I had your boobs!' or 'I'd kill to have legs like you!' We're often very good at complimenting others, highlighting what we consider to be their assets, but we're not very good at seeing that in ourselves. So, if you struggle to put aside your subjective self and look at yourself more objectively, ask someone else! I'm sure a good friend will tell you exactly what they think your assets are.

When we feel clearer on our assets, we can step in front of that full-length mirror and create outfits that look amazing on us.

Activity: Master the mirror selfie

What you need:

your phone

a full-length mirror

Using your phone to take photos of your outfits is another great way to get visual feedback. And taking a selfie in the mirror is a learned skill (don't I know it!).

1. The first trick I recommend to help tackle your inner critic when taking a photo in a mirror is to cover your face. Yep! The logic behind this is that, when you look back at the image, your focus is purely on the outfit (or item of clothing). Simply hold the camera over your face or just take a photo in a way that crops out your head. I guarantee that you'll realise just how critical you were of yourself when your face was in the image, and that's because we tend to look at our face first, outfit second.

2. The second trick to taking an outfit selfie is to pose in the most natural way possible. Think about how you would stand talking to a friend at the park, to a work colleague at the water cooler, or a potential love interest at a party. Think about where you put your hands and the angle of your body, and then, when taking a photo of yourself, see if you can replicate this ease in your body to look as natural as possible. Put a hand in your pocket. Drop one hip. Place one leg slightly in front of the other. *Snap*.

3. Once you've practised your new selfie pose, there are more things you can do: styling! Push up a sleeve. Put your shoes on. Tuck your top in. All these little tweaks can really help to mitigate those negative feelings you might have about how you look and also help concentrate your focus on how an outfit makes you feel.

When you look back at these photos, you'll see someone relaxed, comfortable and confident in themselves and you'll also see yourself as *yourself*! When you take the time to do this, you'll also get a better sense of how you feel because you'll see it in your body language. Feeling good in what we're wearing is intrinsically reflected in how we present ourselves, be it in the mirror or to the outside world. Often when we dislike photos of ourselves, it's our body language that is the dead giveaway.

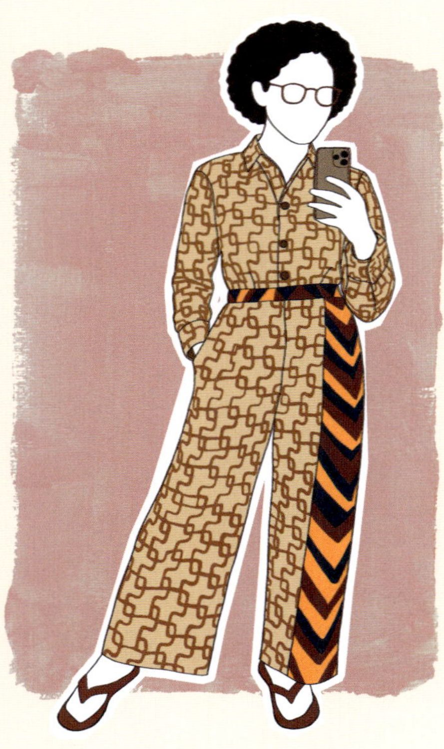

Love yourself, love your style

If you've learnt anything in this chapter, I hope it's that no matter what body you live in or how you choose to cut or colour your hair, style comes from the inside. Having good personal style is nothing to do with your body shape and everything to do with building a superb outfit from head to toe. And that begins with loving and respecting yourself. Sometimes, creating the perfect look can help us access that inner confidence – indeed, that's what this book's all about! – but at the end of the day, loving who you are and finding those special parts about yourself to highlight is the perfect place to start.

What you *choose* to wear is completely up to you, regardless of your body type.

Sometimes, creating
the *perfect look*
can help us access that
inner confidence.

7. DISCOVER THE STYLE BASICS

My top secret to working with the body you have is to know the 'style basics', as I've called them for almost twenty years, and use them to your utmost advantage. These, my friends, are what styling is all about and this chapter contains all my insider styling secrets that I share with every client. They're my non-negotiables and, when you know them and start following them, they'll become your tools for life.

Wear clothes that make you *feel* great

This is my most important piece of advice and, yep, it's that simple. When you feel good, you present yourself to the world in a totally different way.

Does it really matter what anyone else thinks about what you wear? What we choose to wear and what makes us feel good is our decision only. Sure, we can get advice from trusted friends or stylists and seek inspiration (after all, that's why you're reading this book!) but, ultimately, we should only dress to please ourselves. If you enjoy copying a look you see on Instagram, then go for it. If you feel fabulous re-wearing your favourite outfit every week, do it! If you get a boost from wearing head-to-toe colour, wear all the colour you want.

I've had to develop a pretty thick skin when it comes to sharing my outfits on social media. It took me a long time to realise that the people who criticised or critiqued me in a negative way simply didn't personally like my style. And that's okay. But they're not the ones who felt amazing walking down the street – I did. They're not the ones who got a dozen compliments from their peers at a fashion event – I did. They didn't walk into that fashion event with confidence and poise – I did.

If we dress to please other people instead of ourselves, what's the point in having our own personal style? I know ignoring other voices and opinions doesn't come easily – trust me, I'm still learning. But it's an amazingly liberating shift in perspective that we'll dive deeper into in Chapter 9.

Whether the opinion is coming from a partner, family member, colleague or friend, it's time to stop giving in to others and instead be guided by your own thoughts and feelings. It's often the people closest to us who are most brutal in sharing their opinions on how we look, and they can be the hardest people to ignore. But you have to start thinking about how *you* feel, not anybody else. Your tastes and preferences are about what makes *you* happy, not someone else. You are the curator and executor of your own style personality. Absolutely no one else can speak to how you *feel* in your clothes: that's the guidance you can trust.

Trust your instincts

Just as we listen to our intuition when it comes to what we *like* to wear, we should also listen to it when we *don't* feel great in something. If something doesn't feel right – whether it's the fit, feel, colour, shape, style or even price – it's probably not the best choice for you. We all know that feeling when we leave the house and think, 'Oh, I wish I'd worn my favourite red dress rather than this dull black one to meet my date' or 'I should have got changed out of my leggings after Pilates to do the grocery shopping knowing I'd bump into someone from work'.

We can all relate to trying something on in a clothing store and being told by the sales assistant that it looks great but inside we just know it doesn't *feel* right. It's one thing to recognise this in hindsight (and, yes, we all make mistakes we later regret!) but the key is learning to identify them then and there, and letting that instinct inform your decision.

The next time you're shopping and you get told something looks 'amazing' when you don't think it does, try saying, 'Thanks so much but it just doesn't feel like me' or 'Thanks but I'm not 100 per cent sure. There's something not quite right about it'. It's okay to leave a store empty handed, and it's definitely okay to let someone know how you feel, even if you disagree with them. Sometimes we need time to go away and think things through – you can always go back if you decide you do love a piece of clothing. Equally, it's okay to get home and have second thoughts about something you've bought. Perhaps you're not good at saying no (it took me years to not feel pressured to buy something just because I tried it on!) but if you get home and you've changed your mind, that's fine. Sometimes we need to bring items back to our own home to honestly assess them.

Perhaps the patterned blouse doesn't work with anything that you thought it might. Or you realise that you don't have a purpose for the tulle maxi-skirt other than your one upcoming formal event, and the cost-per-wear is unjustifiable. Perhaps the high-waisted jeans look amazing on you first thing in the morning, but you know that once you have something to eat, they're going to feel too restricted around your waist, and you hate that feeling. Or perhaps you simply realise you don't love a new purchase as much as you thought you did when you tried it on in the shop. You take it home, try it on with a few things, think about it, rationalise the cost and consider where it fits in your wardrobe purpose, but your instincts are telling you it's not right, which means it's probably not. These days it's pretty easy to return items, so no harm done! Better to know now than let it sit in your wardrobe, unworn.

Identify what you like about yourself

As covered in the previous chapter, this can be one of the most challenging principles to get your head around. Remember, instead of covering up or disguising what you *don't like* about your shape, identify what you *do* like and focus on that. When you've determined which aspects to highlight, choose clothes that enhance those parts of your body. Starting with the positives rather than the negatives will make getting dressed a much more enjoyable experience, I promise!

Ignore the size on the tag, focus on the fit

We've been ingrained, largely through diet culture, to focus on sizing but I'm sure I don't have to tell you that, in reality, clothing sizes are all over the place. Sizes differ not only from one brand to another but also within the same brand from one item to the next. I've known clients to buy pieces from the same brand on the same *day* ranging from a size XXS to XL!

Beyond all that discrepancy, changes in fashion give us even more reason to deprioritise the size tag. In recent years, clothing has started to be worn in more 'relaxed' ways on the body: the look has become less structured, a bit softer, more oversized. Women, including myself, have started buying clothing in bigger sizes to achieve a look that's both fashionable and comfortable. Imagine that: style *and* comfort!

The easiest way to tackle sizing is therefore to simply focus on the fit that works for you rather than worrying about the size tag. Just like style is personal, so too is how we like our clothes to fit. I appreciate that not everyone reading this will have access to their size from every fashion retailer but if you have found retailers and designers you love and who make clothes for you, this advice applies regardless of your size.

When shopping for myself in store, I often take two sizes of the same item into the changing room and try both on to compare the fit. I ask myself, 'Which do I prefer?' and 'What look or vibe am I going for?' (We'll cover shopping in more detail in Chapter 12.)

A good tailor is worth their weight in gold

When I'm in the changing room, I also ask myself: 'Can I make an adjustment so it fits me better?' And what I mean by that is: 'Can a good tailor make a tweak so this item fits me perfectly?' Being tall, I always check the hem allowance of pants to see if I can take them down and gain any additional length, even an inch. If I try on a pair of jeans and I prefer the more relaxed fit around my thighs and bum but there's a gape at the waist, I know that my tailor can run in the back seam. Everything can be altered for a better fit. Everything. Keep this in mind next time you try on something that is *almost* perfect.

Every item of clothing we buy from a designer or retailer has been designed and fitted on a real person – a 'fit model' – to check the fit and drape of clothing. Fit models are typically chosen based on their body measurements, which are considered representative of the target customer demographic for a particular clothing line. These models are different from fashion models. A fashion model's primary purpose is to showcase clothing in photoshoots or on the runway, whereas fit models are used behind the scenes to ensure that garments fit well and are comfortable for the intended wearer.

Each clothing brand generally has their own in-house model who they use season after season to fit and test their garments. The model works closely with designers, patternmakers and garment technicians to provide feedback on how a garment feels and moves on the body, helping to ensure that the final product meets the brand's standards for fit and quality. This means that when you shop for clothes, every item you try on has been cut to suit the proportions of that brand's fit model. And one designer's fit model will be different from the next. They will be different heights and have different bust sizes, waist circumferences, hip widths and so on. This means that when you go shopping, you are trying on something that has been designed to fit *a* particular person's body type. Yet still, we expect to buy something off the rack that's the 'perfect' fit.

My advice is to stop looking for it! If you're lucky, you'll find it. But if you don't, that's not the end of the world. You just have to keep an open mind and think about any adjustments that can be made to fit your body type. Can the sleeves be shortened? Yes. Trousers lengthened? Yes. Neckline opened? Yes. Waist extended? Yes. Hemline adjusted? Yes. This is why you should find yourself a good tailor who can make simple (or advanced!) alterations to clothing to suit you. While it's an added expense, I personally believe a good tailor is worth every cent. If you don't have one yet, ask around – someone in your friendship group or at work will know someone. And I'm not just talking about getting your 'good' pieces altered. Any item of clothing that does not fit your proportions as you want it to – sleeves too long, waist too big, length too short – will not only look better on you if you have it altered, you'll feel better wearing it too.

What we wear underneath our clothes is just as important

We've talked a lot about the fit of clothing on our bodies, and now it's time to talk about the foundation pieces – our underwear. Here are a few stylist underwear tips I share with clients and follow myself.

Knickers

Your knickers matter! I'm a particular fan of high-rise knickers because they have so many benefits:

- they don't create a line across the stomach

- you can tuck your tops into them – and they'll stay put

- they provide subtle support without the need for full-on shapewear

- they won't create a visible horizontal line across the middle of your stomach under clothes.

My other favourite knickers are seamless. (Seamless + high rise = the ultimate combo!) If you're not a fan of a G-string but want a nice, seam-free look under your clothing, then a knicker with a seamless finish is perfect.

Bras

We're lucky to live in a time where a wide range of bra styles to suit a range of sizes and objectives is available, such as padded bras for those wanting more oomph, minimising bras for those seeking less, convertible bras for multiple styling options and seam-free bras for a smooth line under your t-shirts. Having a range of options in your underwear armoury is imperative to ensuring you achieve the look and feel you desire every day.

Women's clothing is designed with busts in mind, so even something like a jacket is cut in a way that allows for the shape and size of a bust. When the cut, seams and construction of a garment align with your bust, it's more likely to fit you better.

When busts are lifted and supported, regardless of size, your waist will look longer and more balanced. If you have a short torso, this is particularly important if you like to wear higher rise garments. Bra straps should be tightened regularly, even if you have a small bust. With everyday movement and wear (and nature's gravity), bra straps will loosen over time. Every month or so, assess how much you can lift the straps up from your shoulders. If you can lift them to your earlobe, they're way too loose.

Shapewear

Shapewear does a great job of lifting, smoothing and supporting where and when you need it. It doesn't have to be for everyday but then again, why not, if it makes you feel good? If you feel more comfortable and confident wearing tummy support knickers, compression shorts or a padded bra, go for it. Never be afraid to use shapewear to make you feel better.

Rachel's changing shape

My new client Rachel was returning to work after a few years on maternity leave. She was really looking forward to getting back to work and she wanted to make a good impression after being out of the workplace for a few years. Her old work wardrobe no longer fitted well because her shape had changed, and her once-flat stomach that she'd never really thought much about was now causing her a little concern. She needed help finding well-fitting bottoms that she could still wear with all her old work tops.

Rachel loved skirts and dresses for their feminine feel and because she liked to show off her waist. She also didn't shy away from a good pair of heels in the office (which she'd leave under her desk and change into after commuting in her sneakers).

For our session, Rachel brought along her favourite pair of work pumps and we got down to business. I sent her into the changing room with a range of skirts and dresses to try on and she soon emerged wearing dress number one, looking radiant.

I got her to face the full-length mirror and watched her eyes dart up and down her body. They landed straight on her stomach and stayed there. That's all she could see. Her stomach.

What could I see? Her fabulous waist, a balanced silhouette, her stunning blue eyes and her shapely calves poking out from the hemline. Gorgeous.

But Rachel didn't see any of that.

'This looks so great on you!' I said. 'What do you think?'

'All I can see is my stomach,' she replied, as she fiddled with her knickers, trying to pull them up.

'Can I ask what type of knickers you're wearing?' I asked, already knowing the answer she was about to give.

'Oh, some old hipster bikini briefs,' she said, grabbing at them again where they sat underneath her stomach.

It was at this point that we had the 'underwear talk', where I explained how a simple change in knickers – ones that covered her stomach and provided some support – would make a huge difference to how the dress looked on her and how she would feel. Before we finished our session, we purchased some high-rise, tummy-support knickers that made Rachel forget about her stomach and enjoy her new dresses.

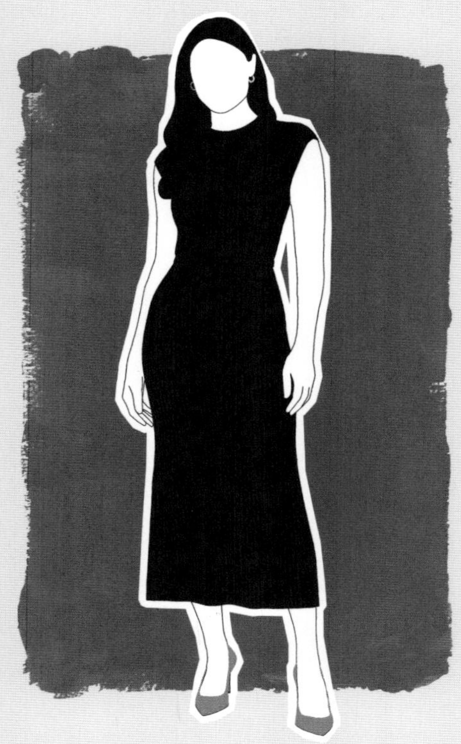

Everything can be altered for a better fit. *Everything.*

Use a full-length mirror – always!

You must always use a full-length mirror when getting dressed. This is possibly one of my biggest non-negotiables when it comes to styling. A mirror is an ally, not the enemy. Just as you find one in a clothing store, it's crucial to have a full-length mirror where you get dressed in your home so that you can properly assess how you look.

It's also important to have enough space to stand back from your mirror – at least 1.5 metres – to provide depth and perspective. Too often we stand so close to the mirror that we simply cannot get an accurate reflection of ourselves. Have you ever taken a selfie on your phone holding the camera close to your face and down your body? Can you picture the odd angle it creates and the imbalance of proportions? That's exactly what happens when we stand close to a mirror. The size and proportions look wrong because the depth of perception is off. Can you see how this can affect how you perceive your outfit when viewing yourself in a mirror?

While many of us despise having to leave the fitting room to look at ourselves in the mirror while shopping, I highly suggest you do – for the reasons mentioned above. The pros will outweigh the cons, I promise.

Using a full-length mirror enables us to objectively critique our outfits to ensure we leave the house as the best version of ourselves, ready to go about our day feeling fabulous. It's also crucial for our ability to build outfits, which we'll explore more in the next chapter.

Spend a few minutes styling your outfit

Many of us think that once we've selected our outfit, we're done. Whoa, not so fast! Once you're dressed, I recommend taking a few minutes to style yourself – this can make all the difference. What I mean here is the 'on body' styling of your outfit: the little tweaks and adjustments that can alter how the outfit works proportionally on your body. Tucking something in, rolling up sleeves, pulling out cuffs, cuffing jeans, unbuttoning and buttoning up, et cetera. And we haven't even accessorised yet!

Merely taking the time to adjust and style your outfit will make it better already. Then you can think about accessories. Does a necklace work or is a chunky cuff better? Or both? A belt? A contrast sock? Or perhaps a knit thrown casually over the shoulders, or diagonally, or tied around your waist. Whatever you choose, the add-ons should complement the outfit but not take away from it.

Ensure you check how your handbag works with the outfit too, especially a crossbody bag, as it can pull at necklines or get caught on buttons. A bag

worn on the body affects your overall look as much as a belt. The wrong bag
can let down the team, whereas the right bag can take your outfit to the next
level.

Styling your outfit in front of a full-length mirror allows you to play with
options efficiently and ensures you can make last-minute changes if
something doesn't look quite right.

Stop critiquing photos of yourself

If I had a dollar for every time a woman said to me, 'I really liked this dress/
jacket/jeans until I saw a photo of myself,' I would be retired and living on
a yacht! (Actually, that's not true, I don't like boats that much. I *would* be
retired though.)

We are so hard on ourselves, particularly when looking at photos. But you
shouldn't be. A photograph is a moment in time. Whether it catches you
off guard or posing in a position you thought was 'flattering', a photo does
not capture the entire story. It does not show how your outfit moved on
your body, how the fabric draped, how it looked from different angles; it
only shows a one-dimensional view of you. And that dimension, may I add,
is also determined by the position and perspective of the photographer.
Trained photographers use this knowledge to frame their shots but most
happy snappers have no idea how much their angles are altering their
subject's profile – unfortunately, often in an unflattering way!

In the same way that where you stand in front of a mirror affects how you
look in it, the angle a photo is taken from can give us a completely skewed
perspective of ourselves. Here's a true story. Many years ago, I met a
professional photographer who had checked out the before and after images
I shared of clients on my website. The first thing he said to me was, 'I knew
you were tall from the angle of your client photographs.' *How did he know
that?*

The photographer noted that my photos were taken from a high angle,
meaning the clients' proportions were somewhat skewed, making them
look longer in their bodies and shorter in their legs. It wasn't obvious to the
everyday eye but it was the first thing this photographer noticed. Being tall,
I was holding the camera at a level comfortable and somewhat natural to
me (chest height), but it was the wrong camera angle for many of my clients,
most of whom are shorter than me.

The fix? Simply to move the camera down and take photos from my waist
height. That helps ensure a realistic, balanced and proportional view of my
subject and, consequently, a more balanced view of an outfit.

The next time you're being overly critical of how you look in a photo, particularly if on the day of the photo you felt absolutely fabulous, think about what I've just said and go easy on yourself!

Style basics are a solid foundation

I hope by now you have begun to develop genuine confidence in your own style instincts. And if not, start practising! As you've learnt, a quick change of underwear and taking a few extra minutes to style your outfit (using a full-length mirror!) can make the world of difference. It may take some effort to change your inner critic, but it is absolutely worth it. If you look hard enough, you can always find something beautiful about yourself; you just have to look with the right eyes and an open heart. Remember, at the end of the day, the only person whose opinion matters about what you're wearing and how it makes you feel is you! If you feel amazing in your outfit, you will show up as your best self. So, dress to impress yourself, not others; so *you* feel great, not to make others look good.

8. LEARN TO BUILD OUTFITS

Style is about putting together head-to-toe outfits that are well balanced, feel right and feel like *you*, regardless of your body type, height, age or size. The secret ingredient to good personal style is how you combine various items of clothing. This is a skill that you can learn – and I'm here to teach you.

Traditionally, we've been taught how to dress individual parts of the body, rather than the whole. We've been trained to focus on making sure we buy or wear the right neckline, the best sleeve style, the most flattering length. But instead, I want you to start thinking about how each wardrobe item works as a team rather than individually. What's the saying in sport? 'There's no I in team.' Let's apply that concept to building outfits too.

How do you want to feel?

This might sound like an odd place to start but I truly believe that the number one key to a great outfit is feeling like yourself, all day. Determining how you want your clothes to make you feel (which you'll learn more about in the next chapter) is one of the key components to building outfits.

How you want to feel, be it relaxed, stylish, sexy or comfortable, will often determine your footwear. As such, your footwear can be an ideal place to start when building your look. I do this often, choosing what style of shoe I feel like wearing depending on how I want to feel on that day for whatever I'm doing. If I'm feeling relaxed, I'll usually choose a flat shoe. If I'm feeling like I want to exude confidence, I'll usually opt for a heel. If I'm feeling in the mood to be bright and colourful, I'll choose one of my bright and colourful pairs of shoes. I suggest you give this approach to getting dressed a try! Once you have a shoe style in mind, you can then choose pieces from your wardrobe that also fit the mood you're in.

Keep in mind that the actual shoes you end up wearing might be determined by the final outfit, and you may try a selection of styles before you land on the right one. For example, if you want a comfy, sporty vibe and know you're going to wear sneakers, you might try a few pairs before you settle on the ones that look best with the rest of your outfit. Equally, you might decide that a dressy flat shoe is what you feel like wearing, and once you've built your outfit around a pair, you might experiment with a few options before deciding which version you like best.

Often shoes are the last thing we put on to 'complete' our outfits, but I want you to start thinking of them *before* you get dressed. Shoes are a crucial piece of the personal style puzzle as they can finish off an outfit with success or failure, so rather than being an afterthought, I want you to prioritise them!

What pieces do you need?

So, you know where you're headed, you know your style personality and you've chosen the type of footwear you want to wear . . . what's next? Do you want to lean into the direction of your shoe – sporty/casual/sexy/professional – or play against them? Asking yourself this can help you decide which other items of clothing you reach for.

Build up from your base

By starting with your shoes, you can now select some 'bottoms' (including dresses) to work with them to elicit the mood you're in and the image you want to project. Perhaps you've chosen some pointed flats and want to show them off with a cropped jean. But then you realise it's too cold for bare ankles, so you decide to swap out the crop for a full-length denim that falls over the shoe, exposing just the point.

Once you've decided on the full-length jeans, you can start to think of tops you can wear. Perhaps you initially try some fitted knits and tuck them in, because you think this will create balance with the longer jeans and flat shoes. But you look in the mirror and change your mind because you don't feel like tucking in and instead select an oversized cotton striped shirt. Over the top you put on a relaxed jumper, pulling out the cuffs, popping the collar and bringing down the hem of the shirt to create some visual interest. Today you feel like being relaxed, comfortable and warm, so this feels right.

On-body styling

We touched on this in the last chapter, now let's go deeper. I'm sure you've all seen some 'styled versus unstyled' videos on your social media feeds comparing a basic outfit with one that's been styled up. What 'styled' means in these examples is how the outfit is tweaked to create a visually cohesive, balanced outfit from head to toe. It's another key factor in outfit building, so let's break it down.

Putting on an outfit is not just putting on an outfit. Yes, you read that right. On-body styling means taking a few minutes to style your outfit – in front of your full-length mirror. You might try tucking in a top, doing up or undoing buttons on a shirt or rolling up the sleeves of a jacket. By looking in a mirror you'll get immediate feedback as to how this kind of styling transforms your look. Perhaps your jeans look better cuffed with your chunky sandals, or your outfit looks neater with your blouse fully tucked in. Perhaps you can achieve the edgier vibe you want with your shirt buttoned up all the way to the top.

On-body styling also includes using accessories to further enhance your outfit. Add a belt, remove a belt. Add a scarf, remove a scarf. Add a statement earring, remove the earrings. Accessories are a great way to add interest and individuality to your outfits but they're not the be all and end all of your personal style. When I meet clients who want to learn how to accessorise, I often say, 'Let's get the basics of styling and building outfits right, and we can worry about accessories later.' Here are some guidelines that can help you style your outfit just right.

Create balance

We all know someone whose style we admire. It might be a friend, a family member, a colleague or someone you follow on social media. These people always look good. You can't quite put your finger on why but something about their style always seems to work.

As a stylist, I can tell you that, chances are, their outfit is balanced. Chances are also that they're not playing by the rules (more on that in Chapter 10!) and that they're using on-body styling techniques to help balance their outfit proportions for their shape.

Show some skin

One of the easiest things to do to achieve balance in your outfit is to show some skin. Now, I'm not talking about excessive cleavage, bare midriffs or shorty-shorts kind of exposure (but if that's your thing, go for it!). Rather, I'm talking about a subtle flash of skin in strategic places, namely ankles and forearms. Yep, it's that simple! Pushing or rolling up the sleeves of your jumpers, jackets or long-sleeve tops to expose some skin at the wrists and forearms can really help to balance the proportions of an outfit. This strategy is particularly useful with pieces that are more relaxed on the body, if you are petite (in height) or if you are feeling overwhelmed with fabric.

If you stand in front of your full-length mirror, hands down by your sides, look at where your elbows align against your torso. This will generally be your 'true waist'. Therefore, when we push or roll up our sleeves towards our elbows, we draw the eye to our waist, and we also create a more balanced silhouette by removing some of the fabric.

Like everything in *STYLED*, these are just ideas to try, to play with, to see how they make you feel. Simply pushing up your blazer sleeves might be your lightbulb moment as to why your oversized blazers never feel 'quite right'. A roll of the sleeves on your favourite floaty blouse suddenly makes you feel less swallowed up by it. Turning up the cuffs on your new pinstripe cotton shirt makes wearing it with your wide-leg jeans feel so much better.

The same principle can be applied to showing off your ankles or even the tops of your feet, which is particularly useful considering the increased popularity of flat shoes and sneakers. When we don't create height or length by wearing a heel, we can often literally feel 'flat' or lower to the ground. This is where exposing some skin at the ankle is a simple yet effective strategy because it creates visual breaks in an outfit, leaving various places for the eye to land. The next time you admire someone's style, check to see if they've applied the 'show some skin' strategy to their outfit building.

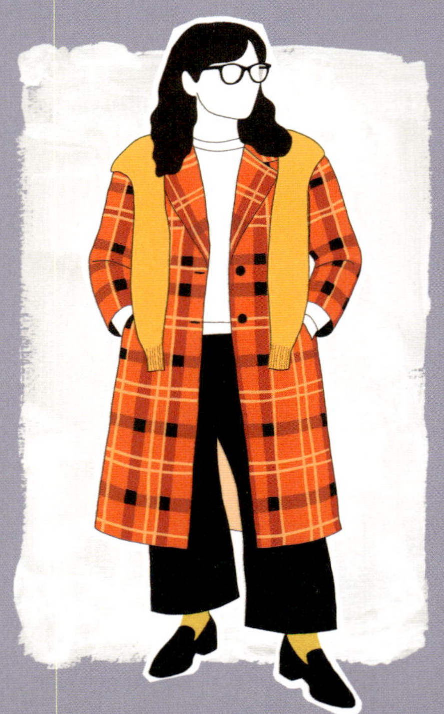

Avoid the awkward in-between

Try to avoid your clothes ending in what I call 'the awkward in-between'. Full-length trousers are intentionally designed to fall all the way to the floor, to achieve maximum proportion and balance. Alternatively, trousers can be deliberately cropped to sit above the ankle bone to expose some skin, to make the proportions feel more balanced. If your trouser leg falls somewhere between these two it becomes an awkward length that is neither here nor there. As we learned in Chapter 7, a good tailor can adjust almost any item of clothing to be the perfect length for you.

Tucking in

Let's talk tucking in! I know and appreciate that for many of you the thought of tucking in your top is both intimidating and fear provoking. Trust me, I've seen the look on many a woman's face when I ask, 'Can you please tuck that in?' The aversion many of us have to tucking in a top is a fear of feeling exposed around the mid-section, especially the hips and stomach. But let me assure you, the benefits of tucking outweigh the negatives in most cases. Let me state my case for tucking in with some examples from my experience of styling thousands of women of all shapes and sizes. Tucking in your top:

- makes your legs look longer

- makes you look taller

- accentuates your waist

- creates the illusion of a waist

- minimises your stomach

- balances your proportions

- creates shape in your outfit

- means you don't have to wear heels.

Did that last benefit get your attention? All of the above (and more) are positive outcomes achieved by tucking in your top. Just like you're learning to embrace your shape, I want you to reap the rewards of 'the tuck'. And there is more than one tuck to choose from!

Any kind of tuck will bring the same benefit to your outfit, be it a full tuck, a French tuck (just the front tucked in) or a side tuck (similar to the French but tucked closer to the hip, on one side or the other). The key to this strategy is to draw the eye upwards to the waist, which helps create shape and elongation.

I've told you why but let's also look at *how*. I've discovered a few techniques that will help you tuck in your top with greater success and mean you stay tucked in!

As I mentioned in Chapter 7, high-rise knickers are one of the key ingredients to a good tuck. Rather than simply tucking your top into your jeans, trousers or skirt, tuck it into your knickers first. Not only can you use your underwear to help smooth out the fabric for a nice, flat finish but your knickers will also help to keep your top in place. Honestly, this is a game changer!

If the thought of tucking in your top concerns you because you feel your stomach will be exposed or accentuated, then another key thing to consider is what you're tucking it into. Just as a high-rise brief will work to your advantage, so too will a high-waisted skirt, pant or pair of jeans. Remember, tucking in a top can create the illusion of a waist if you don't naturally have one. When done right, this can minimise the stomach. A garment that finishes higher on your waist not only helps to achieve this, but it also provides more support to the stomach area. If you've ever worn a low-rise jean, you'll recall having *no* support in the tummy region! But a high-rise jean gives structure and reinforcement to this part of the body.

Speaking of structure and reinforcement, the actual waistband of the item being tucked into is important too. You know that feeling when you put on your favourite pair of jeans straight from the wash, do up the zip and top button, and feel instantly supported? That's the result of good structure, fabrication and tailoring in your jeans, which can be achieved in other items of clothing too. Consider this the next time you go to tuck your top in. What are you tucking it into? Does the item have a tailored waistband or supportive fabric that holds you in? Does it have side pockets that don't pull or a flat front? If it has pleats, do they sit flat on your body? Use your mirror to help you answer these questions.

When doing a full tuck, particularly with something like a t-shirt, blouse or fine knit, I like to finish off with what I call 'the shoulder shrug'. Once tucked in, simply shrug your shoulders up towards your ears to allow the fabric to release and ease just a touch. You don't want too much fabric to blouse over your waistband, defeating the purpose of the tuck but just enough so you don't leave the house looking like Steve Urkel. (Google him!)

Tucking your top in is just one strategy in your style toolbox, one that you can pull out and experiment with day to day. It might not work with every outfit but I guarantee it's a tool worth trying!

Just add one

Another styling strategy that's very useful for outfit building is the 'just add one' approach. It's possibly the easiest thing you can do to elevate your outfit, and I love it because it helps add more interest and dimension.

How many times have you got dressed for an event or occasion only to feel your outfit was a bit dull, basic or predictable? Often, we can get stuck in the literal basics of style and simply choose one item to wear with another, and that's it. A jumper with a pair of jeans, a top with a skirt, a dress with a shoe. Job done. But what if I told you that by adding one more item to your outfit you'll add interest and greater depth, ultimately creating a better look that is both unique and thoughtful?

Consider this scenario: five people turn up to a basketball game wearing the same base outfit of a white boatneck long-sleeve t-shirt, black leather-look jogger pants, leopard-print sneakers and a black bag with adjustable straps. However, they don't all look the same because they've each applied the 'just add one' approach to their outfit. The key is to add something integral to build on the outfit. It's more than just choosing a different-coloured shoe or handbag or a different style of jean, it's choosing an additional item to provide your outfit with more visual interest.

It can be as simple as adding a belt, or a knit over your shoulders (or around your waist), wearing colourful socks or a bag across your body. Speaking of which: when it comes to handbags worn on the body (crossbody or even a bumbag) they become an integral part of our 'look' and should never be underestimated, as demonstrated in these two illustrations. See how different these two women look? Though they share the same base outfit, they have each made the look 'theirs' with a few simple adjustments to on-body styling: different handbags and their 'just one' option – a red jumper versus a puffer vest. Each has a noticeably different style.

The 'just add one' approach is an easy way to 'level up' your style without overcomplicating things or needing to buy something new. My personal favourite 'just add one' item will come as no surprise: a blazer. But it could

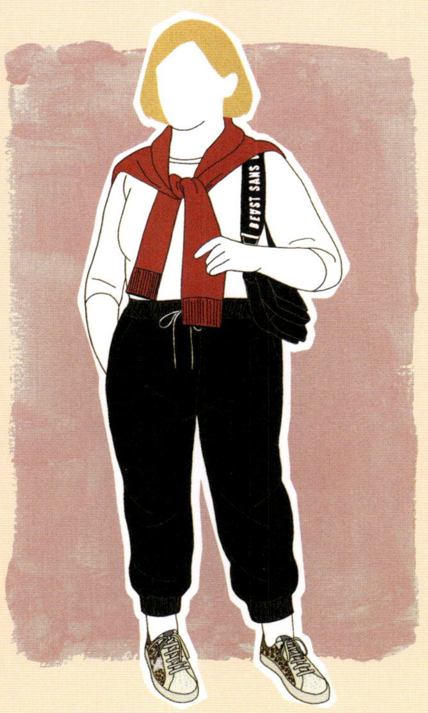

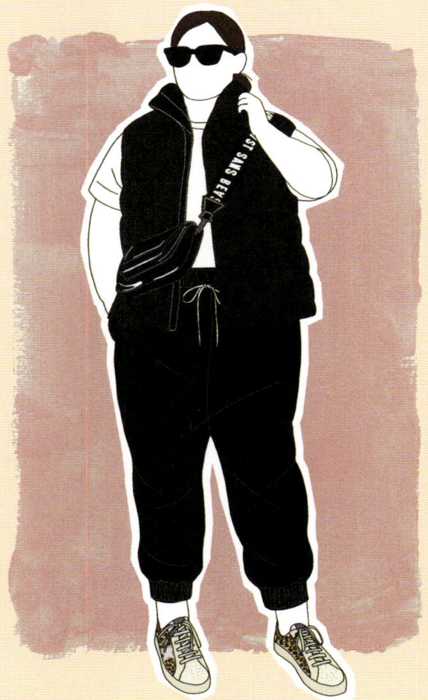

be any form of outerwear (if the weather allows for it), such as a trench, a cardigan, a button-down shirt, a denim jacket, a vest, a waistcoat, a coat, an anorak . . . there are lots of options! Let's look at some more examples of how a variety of outfits can look when the 'just add one' approach is applied.

- Jumper, jeans and sneakers + **crossbody bag with sporty strap**.
- White tank, slip skirt and sandals + **unbuttoned cotton shirt**.
- Blazer, graphic tee, leather trousers and boots + **jumper tied around shoulders**.
- Summer floral dress, tan sandals and mustard woven clutch + **tan belt**.
- Lemon tee, olive green wide-leg pants and cream loafers + **olive green waistcoat**.

You might be wondering if accessories like earrings, necklaces, bracelets, brooches or headbands can be included as your outfit add-ons. For the 'just add one' strategy, I really want you to focus on the fundamental building blocks of the outfit itself. Jewellery is no doubt a great way to inject your personality or a point of difference into your outfit but for this approach let's consider these accessories as the 'salt and pepper' you may or may not add depending on your personal taste.

Focus on how *individual* pieces come together as a whole.

Building outfits while shopping

The importance of building outfits comes into play when shopping too. Unlike how I shop with clients, most of us don't shop for multiple outfits in one mammoth shopping session! We tend to buy individual pieces, one at a time. As a result, it can be difficult to determine if an item will work for us when we style it head to toe with the pieces already in our wardrobe.

To prevent hasty judgements, I encourage you to try things on in your own home. If you're not 100 per cent sure about something (and the store policy allows change-of-mind refunds), take it home and try it on, experiment with it, style it a few ways and make your decision then. Think of an item of clothing like white rice. Without the addition of a few key ingredients, a bowl of white rice is a pretty average meal. An item of clothing can be underwhelming, even average, before it's styled with other things. It's only when the full list of ingredients is thrown in that it brings everything together.

As a general rule of thumb, I would want to have thought of at least five ways to style something new with my existing wardrobe (probably more like ten!). And remember to declassify your items – one piece can often be styled across multiple aspects of our lives. It's just about thinking outside the square.

If you're out shopping but what you're wearing that day does not go with the pieces you're trying on whatsoever, choose another item to try them on with that is similar to something you have at home. Now assess the 'new' item more objectively. Can you envisage this working better now that you're pairing it with leggings/jeans/jumper/sneakers similar to what you'd ordinarily be wearing?

I always ask clients to bring along a pair of shoes that they'd likely wear with what we're shopping for but if you're shopping and the shoes you happen to be wearing don't work with the new item or outfit, then take them off. Better still, if the store sells shoes, try on some more suitable ones to allow you to see the full picture – *the full outfit from head to toe.* You'll be amazed at the difference it makes to your confidence and decision-making.

More than just pieces

Aristotle once famously said, 'The whole is greater than the sum of its parts' and that's exactly what I want you to keep in mind when creating a great outfit. Focus on how individual pieces come together as a whole, rather than the shape, size, fit, length or colour of the individual items themselves. When we focus too intently on the specifics of clothing – a neckline, a skirt length, a leg shape, a t-shirt width – we minimise its potential. Learning to build great outfits is a skill that requires practice, and one I encourage you to persist with. It doesn't come naturally to everyone but with patience, trial and error (and your full-length mirror), I'm confident you'll get there, one outfit at a time!

9. FEEL YOUR STYLE

My only 'rule' is to wear what makes you **feel good**. If you feel good wearing hot pink, wear hot pink. If you feel good wearing skinny jeans, wear skinny jeans. If you feel good showing off your cleavage, show off your cleavage. Honestly, life is too short and already too complicated by the things we need to adhere to. It's empowering to let go of the rules and listen to your instincts.

Clothing can make us feel strong, successful, confident, youthful, sexy, in charge or any feeling we want to express. It can do all the talking without you even opening your mouth. So, let's change the narrative around personal style and, in particular, dressing for your shape. Good personal style is more than what neckline works best for your bust size or what length of skirt flatters your legs. We need to think more broadly about dressing our bodies than what shape of pant will make our bum look smaller (or bigger), what size print suits our petite or tall frame, or what jacket length to wear with a pair of jeans versus a dress.

This might be a bit left field coming from someone who's been repeatedly telling you to look in the mirror, but I would argue that personal style comes down to how you want your clothing to make you *feel* rather than how something fits your body, or even the garment itself. When we listen to our instincts and trust how we feel when getting dressed or trying on something new, rather than only focusing on how we look, we're more likely to make the right choices. Rather than going about our day feeling off, out of place and uncomfortable, we feel relaxed, comfortable and confident. This might mean we mingle at a party rather than standing in a corner, that we might approach someone at the bar and say hi, or that we'll walk into a room feeling confident. We do all of this because we own our style. We know our style. We feel it. It feels us.

When I use the word 'feel', I'm not only referring to it in an emotional sense but a physical one too. How does the clothing feel on our body? When clothing feels comfortable, we often feel more at ease wearing it, and therefore more at ease within ourselves. I'm sure you can relate to having worn something uncomfortable and it ruining your entire day!

Whether you're wearing something that is too tight, restricts your movement, gives you blisters, keeps riding up or down, or feels scratchy on your skin, I guarantee you did not feel at ease. I remember wearing clothing that was too tight for me, leaving me sucking in my stomach all day and, even worse, going without food. Thankfully, those days are gone because I no longer choose to wear anything that compromises how I want to feel.

How does your clothing make you feel?

You've identified the purpose for your wardrobe and have narrowed down the words that describe your style personality. By this point, your style wheels should be in full motion and I hope you're feeling excited about getting dressed and more self-assured and in charge of your personal style.

Now, I want you to think about how your clothing makes you *feel*. It's something we do already, usually subconsciously, but we rarely articulate it. It's often the reason why we go about our day feeling great versus uncomfortable. It's also often the reason we buy something and regret it later.

The simple question to ask yourself is: 'How do I feel in this?' Let's look back at the words you've settled on as your style personality. Those words you used to describe your wardrobe and the images you saved for inspiration are in fact how you want your clothes to make you feel. When you don't feel like this, you won't feel like you. Knowing these words (and referring to them) will help you get it right. You don't have to represent every word of your style personality in every single outfit every day but you should have most of them. Because only then will you feel like you.

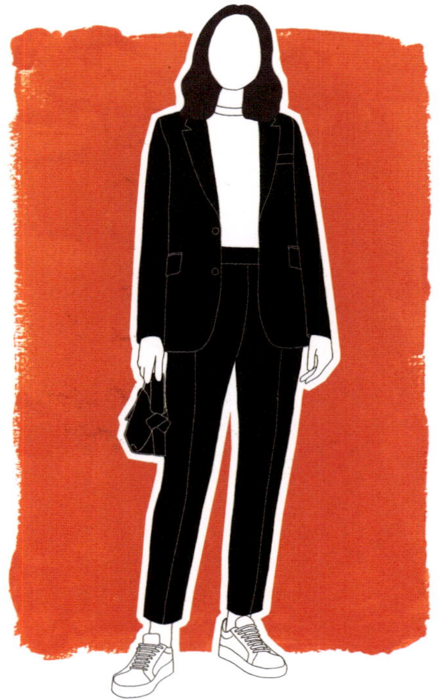

Using a basic outfit – black blazer, black pants, white tee, white sneakers, black bag – as a starting point, let's see how Leah, Sian and I would style it to make it our own.

Sally's style with feeling

My style personality: *tailored, polished, modern, creative.*

When I get dressed, I want to feel these things. Knowing how I want my clothes to make me feel makes it easy to know exactly how I *don't* want to feel. If I were to wear the basic look as shown in the image, I would feel:

- basic
- predictable
- boring
- conservative.

↗ **How I would change the outfit to feel like me:**

- size up one or two sizes in the blazer
- add a graphic tee
- wear a red bag
- add a pointed-toe slingback
- wear a contrast knit over my shoulders
- finish with a pop of red lipstick.

How the change makes me feel:

- creative
- modern
- polished
- cool.

Articulating how the outfit made me *feel* allowed me to make the relevant tweaks I needed to feel more like myself. In this case, by adding more creativity to the outfit and using items that were less predictable, conservative and basic, I changed it up to no longer feel 'boring'.

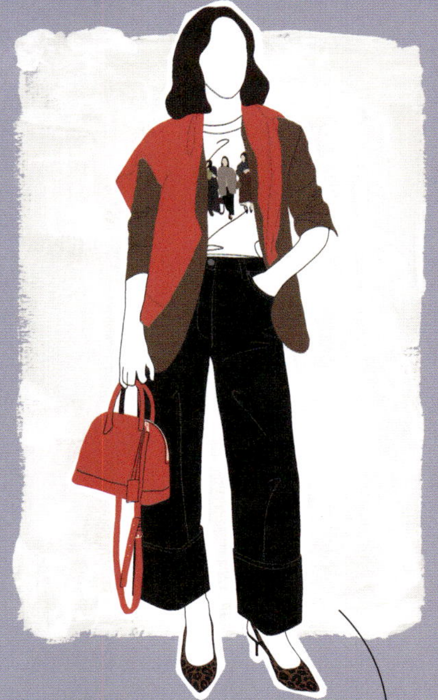

You've seen me wearing this outfit back on page 15. It's a favourite in my wardrobe!

Leah's style with feeling

Leah's style personality: *relaxed, fun, playful, approachable.*

How the basic outfit makes Leah feel:

- restricted
- uptight
- confined
- tailored.

↗ **How Leah would change the outfit to feel like her:**

- change the blazer for a bold-coloured bomber jacket
- untuck the white tee
- add a big earring
- wear a chunky platform-soled sneaker
- cuff the trousers
- wear an old crossbody bag that doesn't match anything.

How Leah feels now:

- relaxed
- fun
- free
- relatable.

If Leah went about her day in the first outfit she simply wouldn't *feel* like herself, and she certainly wouldn't present as the person she wants to be. Her clothing would send a different message to the one she really wants.

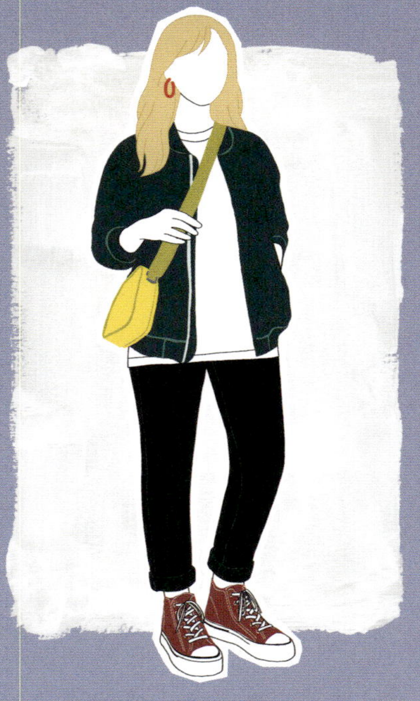

Sian's style with feeling

Sian's style personality: *sexy, edgy, simple, classic.*

How Sian feels about the basic outfit:

- classic (which suits her style personality) but also

- conservative

- boring

- shapeless.

↗ How Sian would change the outfit to feel like her:

- switch out the pants for slim black jeans

- swap the white tee for a fitted black racer-back tank

- roll up the sleeves of the blazer

- add a studded black ankle boot with a heel

- wear an embellished black handbag.

How Sian feels now:

- sexy

- edgy

- cool

- classic.

By leaning into her rocker chic vibe, Sian updates a boring 'classic' look into one that *feels* far more like her. Her embellished accessories lift her monochromatic black wardrobe, giving them the sexy edge that defines her style.

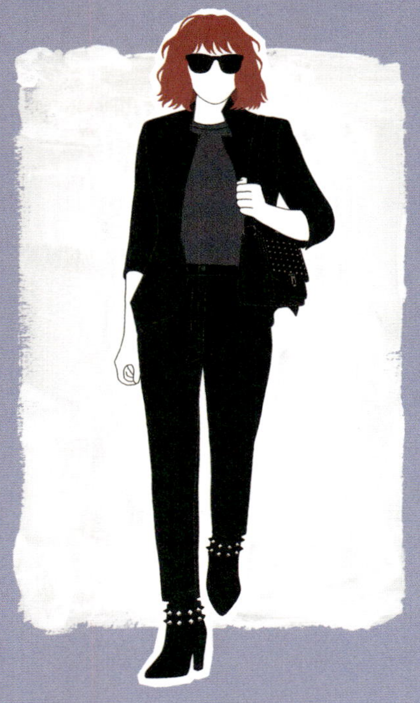

Teaching the 'feelings' approach

As a personal stylist, I've found that teaching my clients to employ the 'feelings' approach to getting dressed and shopping has been a real eye-opener. I think it's always been a subconscious part of my approach but one I probably didn't always communicate as well as I do today.

It's my job to make women feel great through styling them in clothes that look good, fit comfortably and work for their budget. But styling for me has become much less 'transactional' and more conversational. And I love that! To do my job well, I think it's important to hold back from offering my opinion on an outfit when a client first emerges from the fitting room. I want to hear what they think and feel first. Only after they have expressed how they feel both physically and emotionally will I offer my insight into why they might be feeling like this.

This way I am coaching them to trust their own response to a piece of clothing or an outfit, while also drawing out or strengthening the key words that define their style personality. Each time they practise this with me, it strengthens their ability to use this approach – to *feel* their style – and develop the language and a set of questions that help them make sense of that. Of course, as a stylist it would be silly of me to say that my opinions don't count (I'd be out of a job!) but I value my clients' opinions as much as they value mine.

Those thirteen years as a primary school teacher taught me to be a good listener, to read body language, to adapt, empathise and cater for individuals and to not expect everyone to fit into the same box. Being a good personal stylist is also sometimes like being a good therapist! We've all got our own quirks, hang-ups, preconceived ideas, opinions and struggles. And while buying clothes and dressing for your day may hardly sound like the hardest thing in life, for many – women in particular – it can be. My feelings approach has led to some monumental moments in my career. Here are some examples.

Tracey

Tracey is an avid @styledbysally Instagram follower who would always comment on my posts and DM me questions, usually related to body shape. Eventually she booked an online consultation where she had loads of questions about dressing for her shape and height.

Being in her late sixties, Tracey had lots of preconceived ideas about style, colours and body shape. She was inquisitive and on a quest to know the answers to her burning style questions. She needed to know what was right and wrong.

I made it very clear during that consultation that the most important thing was to wear clothes that make you feel good. That's non-negotiable. I also dispelled a few of her style theories, while endorsing others. Tracey told me she felt a great sense of relief and calm after the session because she started to let go of some of those 'rules' she'd been placing on herself and her body.

A few months later, I met Tracey for a personal shopping session. She'd been taking on my advice and styling herself with greater confidence but she needed a bit more reassurance. We entered our first store, a brand she'd admired from afar but had never felt confident to go into, mostly because she wasn't sure it 'catered' for her size and age group. Our eyes both went to the same two blue garments on the rack. It was love at first sight. Before I even had the chance to tell Tracey how much I loved the pieces (and that she should try them on), she asked me, 'Can I wear this?'

Ten minutes later, after browsing the store, selecting a few more things and answering more of Tracey's questions about cuts, fabrics, colours and lengths, we headed to the changing room. 'Let's try on the blue set first, okay?' I said. 'And I'll grab some shoes for you to wear with them. What size are you?'

Tracey came out in the blue shirt and pants set. Our eyes locked, her eyes widening. Then she smiled and walked out to look in the large mirror outside the changing room. I gave her the shoes to slip on and made a couple of tweaks (cuffing the pants and shirt sleeves), then we both looked in the mirror. Tracey put her hand in a pocket and shifted her pose, relaxing one hip. I could tell she felt fantastic.

Tracey did not ask me if the pants made her stomach look bigger, if the relaxed fit made her look shorter, or if the colour suited her. She didn't have to. She felt so good that those questions (or concerns) were not even in her thoughts. Tracey's body language and the words she used to describe how she was feeling – slim, modern and fresh – were all I needed to know.

Veronica

I met Veronica for a wardrobe edit in her home. She was on maternity leave after having her second child, with no plans to return to work for another year or so. Her wardrobe was brimming with beautiful clothes that represented her previous corporate and social lifestyle but didn't really fit with being a full-time mum. Or so she thought.

Veronica was stuck (like many mums) in the 'leggings trap' – wearing her leggings and activewear, all day, every day. While that works for some people, it didn't make her feel good about herself. Comfortable, yes. Confident, no. She used to love clothes and shopping but with less time to herself and a much more casual lifestyle, she'd found herself in a style rut that she was desperate to get out of.

I asked Veronica to tell me how her work wardrobe used to make her feel. 'Confident, competent, stylish, strong,' was her reply. I then asked her how wearing her activewear most days made her feel. 'Lazy, boring, frumpy.'

In that moment, my vision for Veronica's wardrobe was clear. I had to help her to create a style (using her existing wardrobe and a few new, key pieces) suitable for her new lifestyle that would evoke the same feelings as her work wardrobe. Over the next couple of hours, we identified the pieces in her wardrobe that Veronica could 'dress down' for her casual lifestyle. I grabbed her suit jackets and told her to put one on over a t-shirt. I pushed up the sleeves and asked her to show me her jeans. I selected the most casual pair (a boyfriend style), and we added to those with a sneaker. We took a photo.

I then got her to show me her tailored pants. We switched those out with the jeans and kept on the sneakers and t-shirt, then I spotted her denim jacket and asked her to put that on. We took a photo.

I noticed Veronica had a beautiful longline trench which she said she never wore. I suggested that on the days that she had perhaps been for a walk in her leggings, when she had little time to change, was running errands or catching up with a friend for a casual bite to eat, she could wear the trench over her leggings. I threw a knit over her shoulders and added a casual crossbody bag. We took a photo.

We created endless options from Veronica's wardrobe that day and I identified a few things she might buy to help make some of her existing wardrobe work better for her current lifestyle, such as more styles of jeans, a denim maxi-skirt, an oversized bomber jacket and some elevated flat shoes.

Each new outfit we created gave her the same feeling she'd had about her personal style when she'd been going to the office, when she had felt her most confident, competent, stylish and strong. A couple of weeks later, after Veronica added those suggested items to her wardrobe, she sent me the following text: 'I cannot thank you enough for helping me get out of my style rut and back to feeling myself again! I now look forward to getting dressed every day, even if I'm just going to the park or picking the kids up from daycare. I didn't realise how much my self-confidence was being impacted by what I was wearing. You've completely changed my attitude, and I've even felt a sense of increased confidence when interacting with new people. Thank you, Sally!'

Your style, your say

Feeling good in your clothes is the best feedback you can get when deciding if something works for your style. Others may have their opinions but ultimately only you know how you feel, and there's no right or wrong when it comes to that.

But should we take the opinions of others on board? Sure, if they're informed ones. But here's the problem with style: it's subjective. What is good/flattering/worth the money/good value/age-appropriate to one person is not to the next.

As I mentioned, I do offer my own thoughts and insights to clients once they've told me how they feel in an outfit. I'll tell them all the good things, the not-so-good things and how the item fits them, and I'll make suggestions about how to style it and so on. But, ultimately, I will also say that it doesn't matter what I think, it's what *they* think, because they're the one who's going to wear it. I've been in many situations when I have absolutely adored an item or outfit that I've styled a client in. I tell them that it ticks all the boxes, it fits them well, suits their shape and looks fabulous. But if I can tell from their body language or words that they are feeling hesitation and doubt, we'll start a new conversation. It goes something like this:

Sally: Tell me what you're thinking.

Client: I'm just not sure where I'd wear this.

Sally: You could wear it to work with your navy pants, or casually with jeans out for dinner?

Client: I'm not sure about the puffy sleeves. I like the colour and pattern but the blouse feels a bit too feminine for me.

Sally: Okay, let's try this on then. It's a more classic button-down shirt style in the same great colour.

Client: I like this. It feels more me. I can see myself wearing it a lot.

Sally: How do you feel in this shirt?

Client: I feel more modern and sophisticated.

Simply asking clients how they feel puts them in the driver's seat behind the wheel of their own personal style. My approach is to not push or persuade a client to buy something, because the last thing I want is an item sitting in their wardrobe unworn. Sure, sometimes a client needs a little time to warm up to the thought of something that is out of their comfort zone. This is very common. But it's in the conversation that takes place where they verbalise their feelings, that they determine whether a piece or outfit will work for them.

Different ways to wear blue jeans

The same item of clothing, styled in various ways, can elicit a different style and therefore a very different feeling from one person to the next. A classic straight-leg pair of blue jeans that hits just above the ankle bone sounds like a very generic item of clothing, and I'd bet that you own a pair. But even if that one pair was exactly the same wash, cut and brand as mine, we'd style them in a way that reflects our personal style and feels like us. In each of these examples, we are styling the same straight-leg blue jeans in different ways to evoke different feelings:

Modern, edgy, cool: worn with cream pointed-toe ankle boots, olive green longline vest, blue striped collared shirt, brown monogram handbag.

Quirky, casual, relaxed: jeans cuffed to reveal polka dot socks worn with lace-up brogues, waistcoat, t-shirt and canvas tote bag.

Sporty, sexy, casual: worn with a white cropped racer tank, black studded belt, black zip-up hoodie (unzipped), black crossbody bag, sneakers.

Feminine, classy, refined: styled with a floral blouse with a puffed sleeve, pointed-toe heels, cream handbag.

Casual, relaxed, chill: throw on an oversized t-shirt that's side-tucked into the jeans, add a knit the over shoulders, a slouchy shoulder bag and tan slides.

Vibrant, youthful, eye-catching: red trench, blue striped tee, red sneakers, white crossbody bag with contrasting strap.

Using the same basic straight-leg blue jeans each combination reflects a different purpose and individual style and elicits different feelings. What is unique to each are the feelings the complete outfit generates. Age, size, body shape, height and budget are irrelevant.

Looking at these images, see how if we change up the silhouette of the ↗ jeans, switching from straight-leg to other styles, we further emphasise the individual feelings?

Modern, edgy, cool: *barrel-leg blue jeans*, blue and white striped shirt, grey striped knit vest, black oversized bomber, grey patent ankle boots, black quilted bag.

Quirky, casual, relaxed: *wide-leg jeans*, navy and white Breton long-sleeve t-shirt, red bandana around neck, leopard-print flats, oversized basket bag.

Casual, relaxed, chill: *boyfriend jeans,* an oversized t-shirt loosely tucked, weekend blazer, slouchy bag, cap and tan slides.

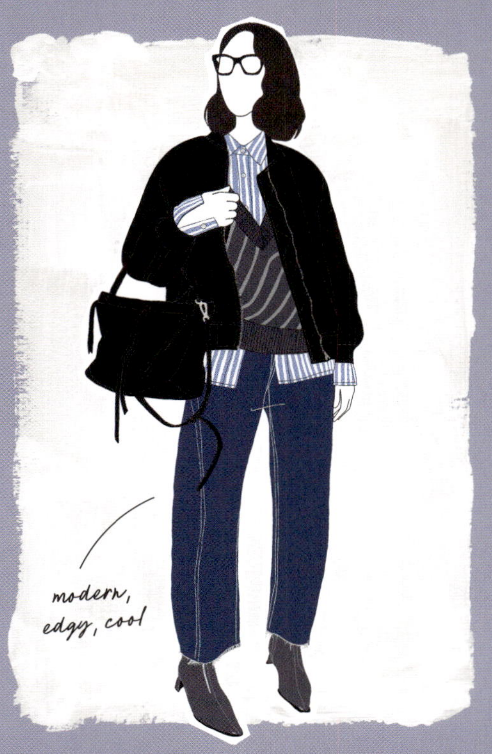

modern,
edgy, cool

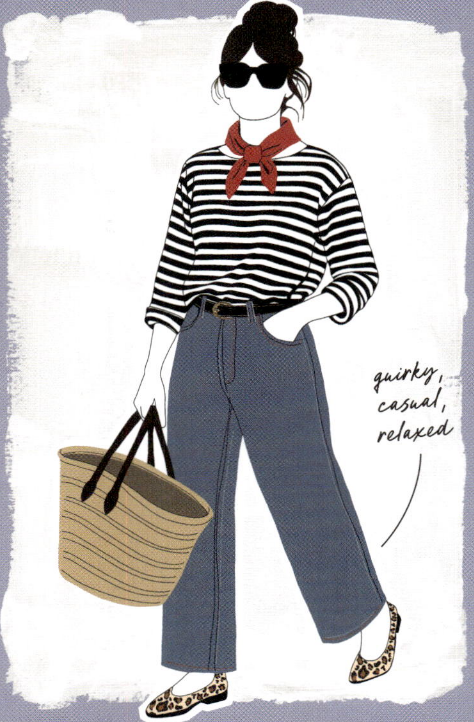

quirky,
casual,
relaxed

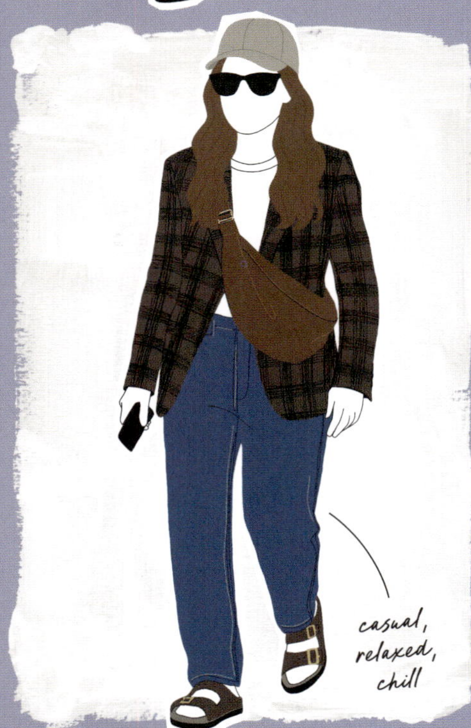

casual,
relaxed,
chill

Feminine, classy, refined: *slim, cropped blue jeans*, floral blouse with a puffed sleeve, pointed-toe heels, cream handbag.

Sporty, sexy, casual: *blue skinny jeans*, white cropped racer tank, black studded belt, black zip-up hoodie (unzipped), black crossbody bag, sneakers.

Vibrant, youthful, eye-catching: *high-rise 'mum' jeans*, red trench, blue striped tee, red sneakers, white crossbody bag with contrasting strap.

Feeling your style when shopping with friends or family

Being able to feel your style can be a valuable and empowering tool when you go shopping with others too. Think of all those times you've been in a changing room, confused by a sales assistant's, friend's or partner's opinion about what you're trying on. Rather than trusting your own instincts, you're overwhelmed by all the voices and input. How empowering would it be to be able to turn around and say, 'I do/don't like this because it makes me feel boring/sexy/conservative/edgy/old/young'? Only you know how you feel – no one else can tell you that. The trick is to pay attention to your inner radar and trust how you feel in these situations, even if you think you might offend someone!

Shopping with friends and family can be fun, rewarding and bonding. But too often I've seen friends and family have what I would consider as too much of a say in what other people wear. As someone who spends a lot of time in changing rooms, I have overheard many a conversation between mothers and daughters, husbands and wives, and groups of girlfriends on a weekend girls' trip doing a spot of shopping. Opinions are flying here, there and everywhere. It's intense! I've witnessed fitting room arguments, tantrums and tears. The situation starts to feel overwhelming, stressful and, suddenly, no fun at all. The shopper – has this ever been you? – feels overcome and confused. They're certainly not having fun anymore.

When you don't have the confidence in that moment to say what you really think, to share how you feel or to disagree with an opinion, you're the one who ends up buying something that you didn't really want to buy or leaving behind something you love.

This used to be me. In my twenties I had a close girlfriend who loved fashion and shopping as much as I did. We'd go shopping every weekend together. We had similar tastes in things and shopped at the same stores. Our shapes weren't too dissimilar either, but she was curvier than me, and not as tall. She also had a lot more self-confidence. Or so I thought at the time.

For years we shopped together, being each other's shopping wing-woman, or should I say 'personal stylist' in hindsight. We'd try things on and share our opinions, positive feedback, encouragement and praise with honesty.

Well, at least that's what I was doing. I never felt as confident as my friend. I would also say never as 'sexy'. But did I want to feel sexy? Not really, that's never been my goal. But because *she* was sexy, and her personality flirtatious, this made me feel 'less womanly'. Having grown up being taller than everyone else, feeling a bit gangly and 'boyish' in frame, I would envy her curves and more feminine silhouette.

On rare occasions, another friend of mine would join us. It was after a few of these shopping trips that she told me my shopping wing-woman was jealous of me. She said this wing-woman's advice was always subjective, highly critical and usually negative. She would put me down, make me feel less confident about my shape and certainly less convinced of my personal style.

My friend felt that my shopping buddy didn't want me dressing better than her and definitely didn't want me looking better than her, so she would sabotage the shopping experience to make me doubt myself and to make herself feel better.

This was eye opening! But guess what? She was right. On reflection, I can now look back and see exactly what was going on all those years ago. Regardless of my friend's behaviour, this happened because I wasn't confident enough in my own personal style and I wasn't confident enough to speak up and express my feelings. Also, I was much younger and still in the process of finding my own style. But that should be a fun, liberating and fulfilling adventure in itself!

I look back on that time as a good reminder of how, as a stylist, a friend, a sister and an aunty, I have an impact on others, and I need to pay attention to how my words come across to others. The advice I give about personal style can impact how they feel about themselves.

Feel into your own style

After reading this chapter, I'm hoping that the next time you go shopping with somebody else or have a discussion with a retail assistant, you'll have the courage and conviction to say what you think. That you'll listen to how you feel and, regardless of the advice you're being given, you'll come to a decision on your own. Thinking about how something makes us feel rather than judging an outfit or a new item of clothing based on how it looks can take a bit of practice but once you start, you'll wonder why you didn't do it sooner. If you can make this a habit, you're more likely to have a wardrobe full of clothes that you love, that you wear again and again, and which bring you joy, confidence and satisfaction.

10. BREAK THE RULES

Many of us love rules. They provide us with boundaries, keep us safe and allow us to live in functioning societies. So even though this chapter is about breaking them, don't get me wrong – rules are not a bad thing. When it comes to personal style, rules can provide us with tools that can help us dress in ways that make us feel most confident. And that's a good thing, right?

When I started my styling business in 2007, I created a document called 'The Rules'. It was a list of dos and don'ts around dressing for your body shape, including advice like 'Avoid front pleats if you have a stomach', 'Don't wear a turtleneck if you've got a big bust' and 'Skinny leg jeans are a no-no if you've got wide hips'. Even writing this now makes me cringe!

I think it's fair to say that back then, these ideas and guidelines appealed to many women when considering their personal style, and when having access to a stylist became accessible to the everyday woman. Clients loved these rules, and so did I. They allowed me to offer my clients very specific advice that was easy for them to implement. If a client had (insert specific body part, i.e. broad shoulders), these were the things they should wear, and these were the things they shouldn't. Simple! It was kind of like colouring by numbers: follow the instructions and voila, you have the perfect outfit.

Over time, though, I began to realise that colouring by numbers didn't allow for much variability, creativity or individuality. As I started to feel less convinced about my rules-driven approach, I realised that intuitively, I'd already begun making changes when working with clients. Instead of telling a client what I thought about something they were wearing or trying on, I was turning the conversation to asking them, 'What do you think of this jean?' or 'How do you feel in this dress?' or 'What do you like or dislike about this jacket?'

I was unwittingly starting to ask clients about how clothes were making them *feel* – my new approach to styling that we covered in the previous chapter. So now I'm going to let you in on a little secret:

There are no rules.
There are suggestions but no rules.
There are ideas but no rules.

There are no rules about what you should or should not wear based on your age, size or colouring. None. Can we adhere to styling principles for our shape *and* wear what makes us feel our best? Yes! If having some guidelines to follow makes you feel like you have greater control over your decisions, be that a specific neckline or colours to wear, then go for it. But if you feel pigeonholed by the rules, then forget them.

I want to liberate you from out-of-date ideas of what you supposedly 'can' and 'can't' wear and show you which styling rules were made to be broken.

Women with big busts shouldn't wear high necklines

The theory behind this advice is simple: high necklines can make women with big boobs look bigger than they are, creating a 'mono-boob' look that appears top-heavy. This can indeed be the case. But let's look beyond a simple neckline and instead look at a complete head-to-toe outfit.

Busty outfit 1

Here our model is wearing a navy ribbed turtleneck tucked into high-waisted wide-leg indigo jeans, a checked camel trench worn open with sleeves pushed up, red pointed low block heels, handbag on the shoulder and a small gold pendant necklace.

Why this works

Wearing navy on the top and bottom means there is no distinction between the upper and lower body and therefore the eye travels freely and easily up and down the body.

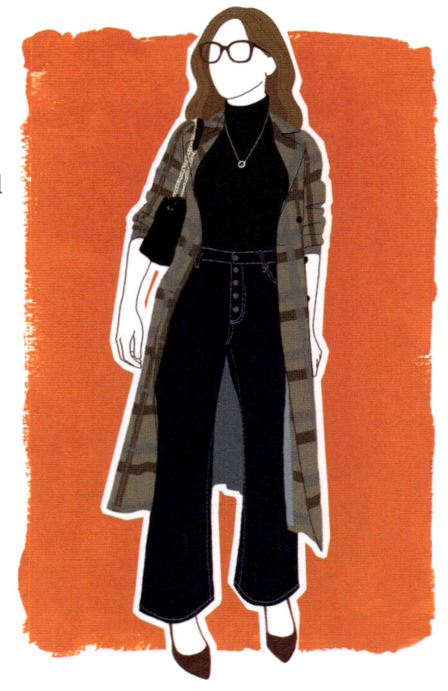

The trench draws the eye vertically down the body. The pushed-up sleeves show a bit of skin, helping to break up the amount of fabric in the trench. The sleeve positioning also draws the eye to the waist, ever so subtly. The pointy toe creates more length through the lower body, as does the small heel.

The shoulder bag nestles neatly in the natural waist where our eye is also drawn, thanks to the pushed-up trench sleeves. The necklace creates a visual break between the height of the turtleneck and the generosity of the bust. The outfit looks proportioned, balanced and fabulous, high neck and all.

Busty outfit 2

Imagine our model now wearing a curve-hemmed white shirt worn buttoned up all the way to the top, sleeves cuffed and rolled, worn over some slim-leg patterned pants, loafers, a top handle bag and knit tied loosely over the shoulders.

Why this works

A collared shirt buttoned all the way to the top looks chic and polished, regardless of one's size or shape. The buttons draw the eye to the face and frame the outfit. The curved hem of the shirt creates a soft drape, not a hard horizontal break between shirt and trouser. The curved hem also draws the eye up to the hip on either side of the body, making legs appear longer. To balance out the buttoned-up shirt, sleeves are rolled and cuffed to approximately elbow length. Remember, when we roll or push up our sleeves, we subtly draw the eye to our waist. A rolled sleeve can also make a shirt look more interesting, simply because it adds a further element of styling to your outfit.

With the patterned trousers, there's a nice synergy between upper and lower body, again leaving the eye to travel seamlessly up and down, creating a harmonious line. The trousers hit the ankle bone, so that when worn with loafers we see just a touch of skin where, for most women, will be the narrowest part of their lower legs.

The final touch is a light knit thrown over the shoulders and tied to sit in the decolletage, adjusted slightly to sit off-centre. Grab a top handle bag (of any size) and place over the arm to create another visual point of interest away from the bust area. The full outfit is proportioned and balanced, and looks fabulous, high neck and all.

Maya's new approach to dressing

I met Maya for a home styling session to help her make better use of the clothes in her wardrobe. Like many women, she had plenty of clothes but was wearing only 20 per cent of them on high rotation, while 80 per cent gathered dust.

Maya was average height, with narrow shoulders and a generous bust. She was a conservative dresser but liked to show off her curves, so had a wardrobe full of wrap dresses and wide belts. She also loved to wear high-rise jeans with her t-shirts tucked in, a styling tool she employed to show off her waist when she wasn't wearing one of her dresses. She'd invested in a few blazers but every time she put them on they just felt wrong, yet she couldn't put her finger on why.

I asked Maya to show me how she'd been styling them by putting together an outfit from her wardrobe and telling me exactly what was feeling 'off'. She got out her favourite white jeans, adding a tan belt and ankle boots, her favourite navy tweed blazer and a white V-neck t-shirt.

I asked Maya, 'Do you have any crewneck tees or tops?' She went to her wardrobe, had a flick through, opened up her drawers and came back and said, 'No, all my tops are V-necks.'

'I think you need some crewnecks!' I said.

'But I didn't think I could wear a high neckline with my big bust.'

'Yes, you can!' I said. 'A crewneck works perfectly under a blazer – let me show you.'

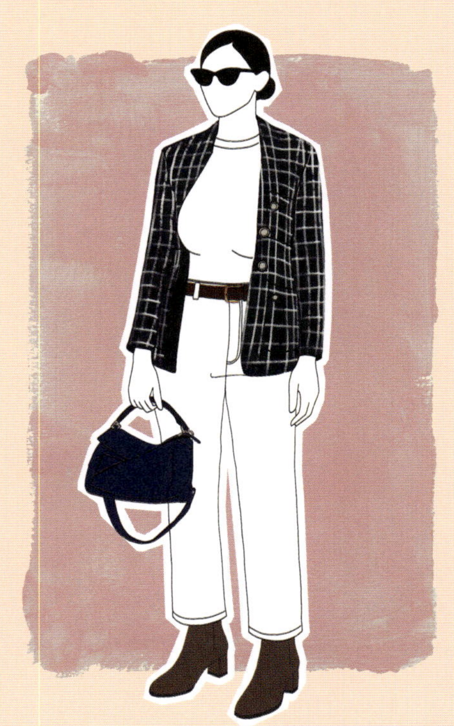

Maya could wear a high neckline with her generous bust for many reasons:

- most importantly, she felt good in one

- the high neckline added polish and modernity under the blazer

- the blazer colour looked amazing on her

- her blazer accentuated her shape because of its tailored cut

- the crewneck top was tucked into her jeans

- her jeans sat high on her waist, visually her narrowest point

- the added belt drew the eye to the waist even more

- Maya's outfit was balanced.

Maya had been following rules that narrowed her choices when it came to buying clothes for her shape. She was hung up on a simple neckline rather than thinking about the complete picture, which included how she was feeling in her clothes. When Maya shopped she was discounting anything with a high neckline, which presented numerous challenges for her, particularly when her favourite brand rarely designed a neckline other than a crew, boat or turtleneck.

After showing Maya how different her outfits looked with the simple change of a neckline (I simply asked her to wear her tops backwards for the exercise!), she couldn't quite believe it. Letting go of this 'rule' gave Maya so many more options. Sure, a high neckline can accentuate a generous bust but first you need to ask yourself:

- Do you mind accentuating your bust?

- What's the colour, fit, fabric, shape of the high-necked item?

- How are you styling it?

The answers to these questions will be different for everyone depending on tastes, preferences, body confidence, personal style and body proportions. How someone with a big bust *feels* in a high neckline is ultimately the most important factor.

Petite women cannot wear long skirts and dresses

Styling folklore has it that skirts and dresses that fall below the knee will make a short-statured woman look shorter. Can this happen? Yes. Is it a 'rule' that applies regardless of how said petite woman styles her long skirt or dress with other items from her wardrobe? No.

Petite outfit 1

Here our model wears a tiered midi-skirt, a scoop neck singlet tucked in, a relaxed blue denim jacket with sleeves rolled, ballet flats and a crossbody bag.

Why this works

The midi-skirt is being worn on the waist, not the hips. The skirt falls to above the ankle bone, not on it. The t-shirt is tucked in, not untucked. The crossbody bag sits above the hip, not on it.

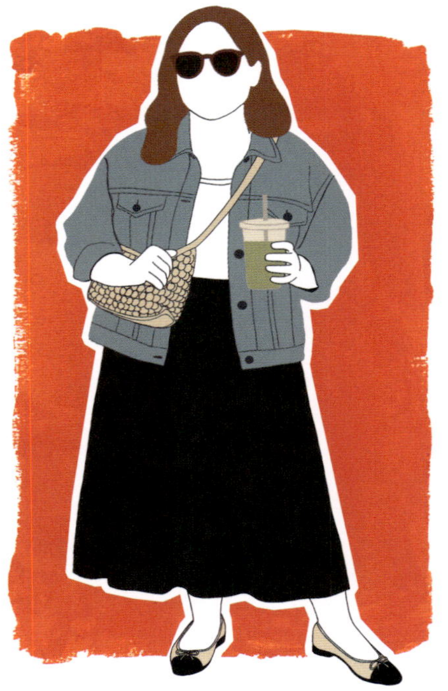

Despite someone being petite (officially that's under 162 centimetres), they can create the illusion of height simply by wearing things on their natural waist. When we wear items on our waist such as a belt and/or a crossbody bag (and tuck our tops into them), the eye is drawn up the body to this point, meaning the legs look longer. When a skirt falls a couple of centimetres above the ankle bone, we create balance because they are not drowning in fabric. A petite woman will not feel short when the proportions are right.

Flat shoes (ballet flats are good because they expose even more skin at the ankle, creating more visual length), a denim jacket of any style (neat/oversized), with its sleeves pushed up for bonus points, and a crossbody bag finish off the look. By sitting the bag somewhere between the waist and hip, it's technically falling on the upper body and therefore drawing the eye up. When a bag hits below the hip we're drawing the eye down the body.

Petite outfit 2

Now, imagine our model wearing a high-necked summer maxi-dress that falls (gasp!) all the way to the floor, flat sandals, a woven basket bag and sunnies.

Why this works

The dress falls all the way to the floor – a true maxi. But never fear, the dress has some strategic design elements that make it work, even with flat shoes. The neckline is high and the dress is sleeveless, with a cutaway design at the shoulders. The extra skin on show elongates the arms and draws the eye to the shoulders making them appear broader, while the extended fabric of the high neck makes her appear taller and narrower.

There's an ever-so-subtle seam on the waist, drawing some attention to it. From this point, the dress falls beautifully to the floor in a slight A-line shape. While the flat summer sandals are not adding any additional height, this is not required because the eye is drawn up naturally to the shoulders and to the seam at the waist. Additional items like a fabulous necklace or earrings, a belt, sunglasses or a pop of lipstick all help to once again draw the eye up.

If you feel pigeonholed by the rules, then *forget* them.

'I can't tuck my top in because I have a tummy'

This is often more a personal fear than a prescribed rule but nonetheless it's a common worry and one I've helped many women overcome. One tactic I use when showing clients how to tuck in their tops for the first time is to style them in head-to-toe similar colours, i.e. a tonal look. It can be any colour – navy, grey, hot pink! – and not just 'slimming' black. Wearing the same or similar tones of a colour, including prints and patterns, from head to toe, draws the eye vertically up and down the body rather than breaking the body into two distinguishable parts, causing the eye to land on the mid-section.

The most important element of this outfit is the pants. A pant that is 'tuck-in-able' will do all the hard work for you, supporting your stomach much like a good pair of high-rise or tummy support knickers. They should have some structure to them, preferably tailored, meaning they have a waistband, pockets and a front zip, and are made of a fabric with some weight and minimal stretch that glides, drapes and falls on the stomach. Rigid denim is a good example compared to denim that's full of polyester and spandex. Other good fabrics for support and ease are wool and wool blends, mid to heavy cottons and some manufactured fabrics like viscose.

Why do we also want tailored elements like pockets and a front fly, possibly even some pleats? This is all about distraction. These design details help to break up the area and therefore minimise the appearance of the stomach. Pleats on trousers can help too but not always. A well-made and well-positioned pleat will sit nice and flat, provide a nice distraction and even offer a little more 'wriggle room' for the stomach to sit (or hide) under. However, a poorly placed and poorly made pleat will add additional bulk to the area and should be avoided. Pleats are tricky but just because you carry your weight in your stomach doesn't mean you can't wear them.

Cuddly tummy outfit 1

Here our model is wearing a puffed-sleeve, scallop-collared pink gingham blouse, tucked into a mid-blue denim maxi-skirt, red belt, white and red sneakers and red crossbody bag with a thick strap.

Why this works

As mentioned, denim is a great fabric to tuck a top into because its sturdiness and structure helps to support the stomach area. The scallop-edged collar worn fully buttoned draws the eye up to the face, as does the bright pink pattern worn on the upper body. The full sleeve of the blouse creates additional width up top, helping to add stature and impact.

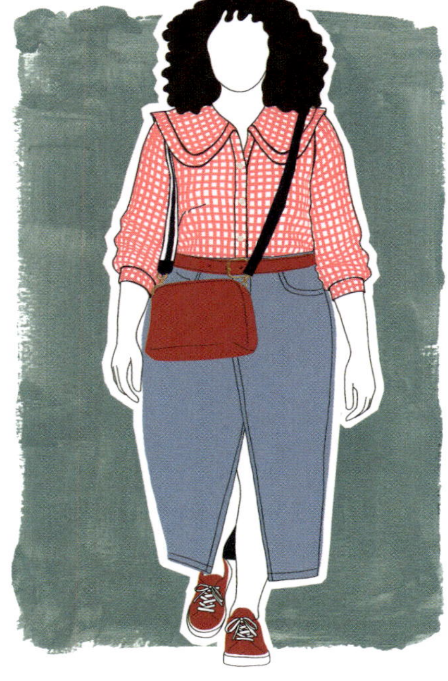

Adding the belt draws the focus up to the natural waist and away from the stomach. The bag worn across the body and nestled on the hip also assists in drawing the eye up, maintaining all the focus on the upper body.

The long denim skirt creates visual length on the lower body, which also minimises the stomach. The accessories work together to create a harmonious and complementary colour palette, resulting in a well-balanced and styled outfit from head to toe.

Cuddly tummy outfit 2

Now, imagine our model wearing navy wide-leg, cropped trousers with a lilac crewneck knit tee (fully tucked), navy blazer, navy belt, two-tone slingbacks and cream handbag.

Why this works

This outfit employs the 'third piece' method. A third piece can be a jacket, blazer, trench, vest or cardigan that you add to the outfit, which are all a great way to 'cover up' the stomach area and help you feel more comfortable when tucking your top in. Adding a jacket won't 'ruin' the look or defeat the purpose of the tuck at all, because even when we add the third piece, we can still see the tuck underneath. This is why we wouldn't button up our jacket in this instance, and why I discourage you from positioning your third piece items *over* your stomach (a very common strategy I've seen employed by thousands of women over the years). It's important to let the third layer sit open on the body so that what you're wearing underneath, i.e. your fabulously tucked-in outfit, can be seen and appreciated. And you'll get the added bonus of the third piece creating vertical lines up and down the body, dividing the body into thirds, and visually minimising the stomach. Voila!

The rule I learned to break

Is there a 'rule' you've been adhering to when it comes to dressing for your shape and proportions that we can also challenge? Let's find out! I'll share mine first.

***Rule:** small busts should avoid shapeless clothing and instead wear fitted tops to enhance the bustline.*

I followed this rule for many years. I'd choose fitted tops like tanks, turtlenecks and t-shirts made of stretchy fabrics that supposedly made my boobs look bigger. I'd generally balance them out with a wider bottom, like an A-line skirt or a bootcut jean.

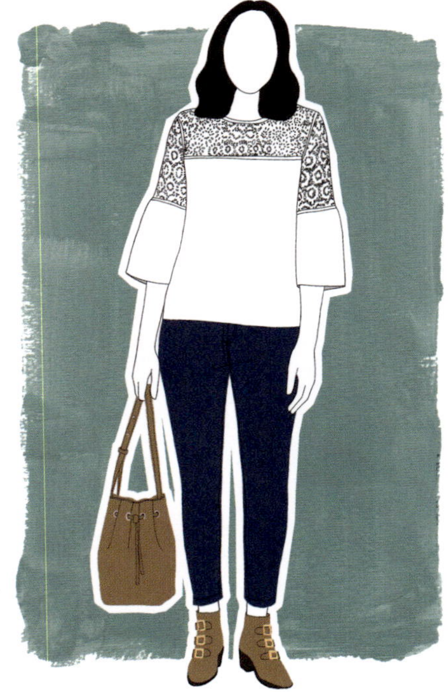

Then skinny jeans came in, and I didn't like that my 'skinny' tops suddenly felt too fitted when worn with a much tighter jean. I didn't feel balanced and, importantly, I didn't feel like myself. Wearing fitted tops with skinnies (especially low-rise), I felt very self-conscious about my body, especially my mid-section. I felt exposed more than anything else but I wasn't sure what I was supposed to do.

Around this time, 'babydoll' tops came into prominence. Typically, these are fitted around the bust and then flare out from the waistline. They can be sleeveless, short-sleeved or long-sleeved but the bodice is characterised by its loose, flowing design.

When I first tried on this style, knowing that it was going against 'the rules', I worried that I would look shapeless and more flat-chested than I already was, because there was more fabric than I was used to wearing on my upper body. But when I teamed it with my skinny jeans, I realised that, actually, the babydoll style looked really good on me! It looked good because I felt good. While it didn't 'enhance' my bustline, it did work with the slim proportions of my skinny jeans. I felt *balanced* from head to toe.

The fact that I wasn't enhancing my bust didn't concern me, because I was now looking at an outfit that felt new and fresh and was, in fact, creating a new silhouette for me. The skinny jeans helped to enhance my long legs, something I'd never done strategically, and ironically the less-fitted top made me feel more confident because I wasn't feeling like I had to suck in my stomach all day! Had I been stringent in following the rules and not tried something new, I wouldn't have felt as good in skinny jeans.

Okay, now it's your turn to break the rules!

It looked good because *I felt* good.

Activity: Break the rules

What you need:
pen and paper

I want you to think of one style or body shape rule that you've learnt, read about or been told, and let's challenge it right here and now.

1. First, write your chosen rule down.

2. Now, think of an item of clothing that goes against this rule (this may be something you already have in your wardrobe or something that you don't own because you don't think it suits you).

3. Next, write down as many ways you can think of to style this item with your current wardrobe.

4. Finally, wear one of these outfits ASAP (if you don't own it, go to a shop and try it on)!

Note that I stipulated wearing the *outfit* and not just the item. Assessing how you feel in any item of clothing should be based on how that item comes together within the context of the complete outfit.

Be a rule breaker

Fashion and style have come a long way since I started out as a stylist. Thank goodness! No longer are we bound by silly rules that have no place. If anything, stylish women are identified by how courageously they defy them! So, embrace this newfound era of self-expression and have fun playing with creating and breaking style patterns. Use the old commandments as a springboard for new ideas . . . Petite figures: drape yourself in material. Long legs: crop your suit trousers. Business attire: mismatch patterns and add a 'wrong shoe'. Such brave moves have created new style 'theories' over recent years – perhaps yours will be the next big trend!

My objective with
this book is to
make personal
style *easier* for you,
not harder.

11. DISCOVER YOUR COLOURS

This chapter might ruffle a few feathers – but it might also free you from any long-held confusion around 'colours'. I find it liberating but I must be honest: my position stems from my own biases. I'm not a colour consultant and I personally find colour theory and analysis confusing – warm versus cool, summer versus spring . . . How do you really tell? So, I choose not to buy too much into colour theory and analysis. When it comes to personal style, I find it limiting and unhelpful.

If you haven't heard about it, colour analysis is used to determine which colours flatter you most, based on the colour of your eyes, hair and skin. On this determination, a season and accompanying colour palette is designated to assist you with choosing the 'best' colours to flatter and suit you. If you're someone who has had your colours done and this approach works for you, that is totally okay – no judgement here. But I know for a lot of women (me included), the idea of a specific palette of colours that suits us – or doesn't – is more hindrance than help in many situations.

My objective with this book is to make personal style easier for you, not harder. In the same way I encourage you to dress to please yourself, wear what you feel good in and trust your own instincts, I suggest taking a similar approach to choosing colours. To keep things really simple: if you've been wondering about what colours to wear and which ones to avoid, the answer might already be sitting in your wardrobe.

Activity: Know your colours

What you need:
pen and paper
your phone

It's time for another practical activity. Get out a pen and paper or open a notes app on your phone. Now, go to your wardrobe and answer these questions:

1. What colours do you see most of?

2. Of these colours, which do you feel great in?

3. Can you write three reasons why you feel great in these colours?

4. When you wear these colours, do you receive compliments from others?

5. When looking at the colours you like most, are they mostly for upper body or lower body items, i.e. tops or skirts? (Dresses and long jackets are considered top of body.)

6. Are there any colours in your wardrobe that you don't wear much?

7. Can you write down three reasons why you don't wear them?

Your answers will be the starting point to determining the colours that work best for you. The colours that you identified in questions 1 and 2 are colours that you instinctively feel your best in. They're colours that you love, that you're drawn to when you go shopping and that you find easy to wear. They're probably also the colours that actually look good on you! When you put them on and look in the mirror you see your eyes light up, your complexion brighten and your smile widen. They're *your* colours – but they're not your *only* colours.

I should also say that if black is one of your most worn colours, that counts too. If black is the colour you invest in and feel great in, then black is one of your colours!

Colour preferences

When we think of our favourite colours, we may have a preference for a particular shade. For example, when I open up my wardrobe it's clear that green is a clear favourite of mine. I have jackets, knitwear, shirts, pants, dresses and even shoes and bags in green. But when I put all of those green pieces out onto a rack, side by side, something becomes very obvious.

There are particular shades of green I have more of – the most prominent being somewhere between a mid-green and dark green, and mostly in more muted shades rather than bright ones. If I narrow this down even further, I can see that my preferred greens are sage, olive, forest and moss. There is not much mint or true emerald green, though I have dabbled in both. When I think about these pieces more closely, I can identify another interesting fact. The items in shades of green I love most are pieces I invested more money in. The less-preferred shades I spent less money on.

Case in point, a mint green vest and trouser suit I bought from Zara during the pandemic. I still own it because it's a great cut and I had the hem on the trousers taken down for the perfect fit. When I first wore this suit out of the house to work (i.e. not just styled for Instagram), I took a mirror selfie while waiting for a client in the changing room. I could immediately see that I looked a bit washed out, a bit 'meh'. It needed a lift. So, the next time I wore it, I changed a couple of things. I wore a crisp white shirt underneath the vest, meaning the pale mint was not closest to my face, and I wore a bright lipstick. Problem solved.

A few years later, I bought a similar coordinating vest and trouser, this time by Tibi. The colour was described as 'hazel'. It looked incredible the minute I put it on, wearing minimal make-up and my everyday Chanel 'nude' lippy. This shade of green didn't need any help. And guess what colour my eyes are? Hazel.

The truth is that you *can* wear every colour but you will have natural preferences towards certain colours, shades and depths that work best for you.

The power of make-up

When you wear a colour close to your face, you are likely to immediately love it, loathe it or feel ambivalent about it. But any hesitation does not necessarily mean it's wrong for you, because there's something we all have at our disposal that can make all the difference when it comes to wearing colour: make-up.

Just like the history of clothes, the origins of make-up are also quite fascinating! Make-up has been worn by both women and men for all sorts of reasons, from cultural to religious and from an expression of one's individuality to conforming to the fashion of the day. But the reason I bring up make-up here is that it has the ability to transform our faces in ways that allow us to wear more colours. And it doesn't have to be a lot of make-up! Think about a simple brush of mascara, a dab of blush, a pop of lipstick, a touch of undereye concealer. We can use make-up to our advantage, helping take a colour from looking a bit drab to fab.

Because we tend to wear make-up on our faces (mostly), I want to talk specifically about the colours you wear next to your face, 'top of body'. Why? Because your face is where people look when they meet you. When you look in a mirror to assess if a colour 'suits' you, you judge that by how your face looks.

What about the no make-up readers, I hear you asking? Don't worry, I'm here to make it easy for you too. If you wear no or minimal make-up, then ensure the colours you wear closest to your face are *always* your best colours. These do all the work for you. Unlike the rest of us who can manipulate our faces with a little bronzer here, an eyebrow pencil there, you need your top-of-body colours to complement your natural features. How do you do this? Let me show you four ways. PS: This advice applies to those of us who do wear make-up too, and you may even find that you don't need much make-up if you keep these ideas in mind!

Enhance your eye colour

Select colours that enhance your eye colour. I mentioned that one of my preferred shades of green is olive and my eyes are hazel. When I wear olive green, I know I can wear less make-up because olive brings out my green eyes, and I look and feel good.

Avoid matching your skin colour

Remember Carrie Bradshaw's 'naked dress' in *Sex and the City*? The dress was exactly the same colour as the actress's fair skin, so she looked naked. Now, wearing the same colour as your skin tone is tough to pull off at the best of times but when you don't differentiate your skin from your clothing using make-up, you're going to look bland, washed out and, as Carrie famously described, naked.

Wear colour, not neutrals

Not only will your 'naked' colour wash you out without make-up, so too will other shades of neutrals such as beige, stone, taupe and cream. When you don't wear make-up, these colours are much harder to wear near your face. Your preferred colours will be so much better on you than any shade of beige.

Add textural interest

Have you ever put on something shiny or shimmery and noticed how the light reflects on your face? This can be really helpful when you want to ensure your clothing 'lifts' your face rather than dulling it. Fabrics like satin, silk, velvet and leather, or textures like fluffy wool, metallic, sequins and patent all help to create interest and highlight your gorgeous make-up-free face.

The truth is that you *can* wear every colour.

Colours and age

When I meet clients who've had their 'colours done', it's important that I ask them when. If they tell me it was over twenty years ago, it's time to have a chat! As we age, so many things about us change: our lifestyles, our jobs, our personal style, our bodies, our hair and complexion. The colours that used to 'suit' us in our twenties, when we may have had a tan (real or fake), when our hair colour may have been natural and when our skin was likely more evenly textured and plump, are very likely not the colours that suit us today. They may not even be the colours we like!

Nothing ever really stays the same. Can you imagine wearing the same outfits you wore when you were a teenager? The same heels you wore to the office now that you're semi-retired? The same trends you tried in (name any decade!)? When you stick to the same colours for your whole life because you were deemed an 'autumn' palette in your twenties, you may well find those colours don't suit you anymore now that your hair is grey or shorter, or you no longer wear much make-up. Or, you simply prefer different colours these days. As such, it's important to continue to evolve your wardrobe hues along with the rest of your life.

One of the most significant transformations that most women experience is their hair changing colour – notably, going grey or white. The importance of hair colour should not be dismissed as it will change your overall look in an instant. Your hair colour and how it complements your outfit can be the difference between looking amazing or blah. Just as with make-up, we have some control over this. I like to think of hair colour and style as equal in significance. Hair frames the face. It can bring warmth and softness to our skin tone. It can also create a jarring contrast. Consider olive skin and caramel highlights (soft contrast) versus fair skin and jet-black hair (high contrast).

This is why, if you embrace the natural process of ageing and go grey, you may need to rethink your colour choices. It doesn't mean it's time to throw out your entire wardrobe of pastels and instead start buying deeper colours but it might mean you re-think your make-up or colour combinations to work better with your new grey hair.

Bev updates her colours

When I met Bev, she was in her late sixties and recovering from chemotherapy treatment, which had resulted in the loss of her hair. She had been colouring her hair all her life but post-treatment she had decided to embrace her natural grey as it grew back and put her salon costs towards a styling session with me, because she wasn't feeling great about her wardrobe.

She told me she had been deemed a 'deep warm' when she'd had her colours done in her thirties. I asked her what colour her hair was back then, and she said she'd always been a natural brunette and up until her treatment had continued to dye her hair dark brown. She opened her vast wardrobe of beautiful deep, rich tones of purple, burgundy, forest green, chocolate brown and lots of black. These were all colours Bev had been told were her 'best colours', the ones that had dictated every purchase in the last thirty years.

I asked Bev how she felt wearing these colours today. 'They feel too heavy. I look in the mirror and I feel washed out,' she told me. With her new hair colour and a paler skin tone (she didn't go in the sun anymore), Bev found her wardrobe didn't work for her as well as it used to, because Bev wasn't who she used to be, thirty years earlier.

Taking all the beautiful, deep hues from her wardrobe, I showed her how to 'lighten up' her style by adding some softer tones like crisp white, baby blue, lemon and soft pink. These new colours, when paired with her existing ones, created a softer look that made her wardrobe – and Bev – come to life. When Bev looked in the mirror, she commented that she felt 'fresh', 'happy' and more 'alive' in her new colour combinations. She realised that she'd discounted so many colours she really loved and was naturally drawn to because they weren't considered to be right for her.

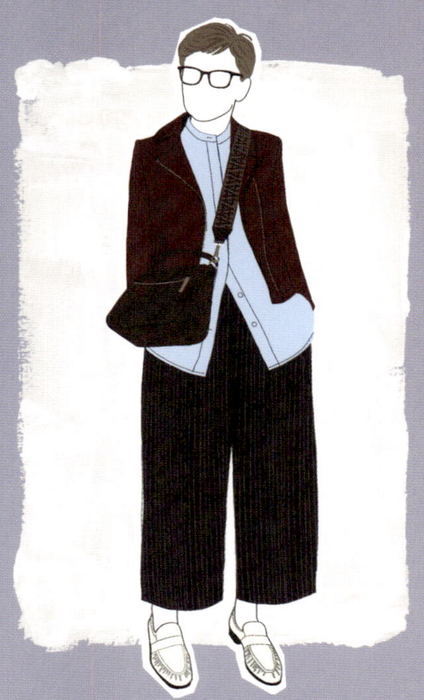

Redefining neutrals

You've probably read advice that your wardrobe should contain some neutral building blocks – after all, that's what we see in endless Instagram reels and flat-lays, right? When you think about neutrals, what usually springs to mind are basic black, navy, white, grey, tan and so on. And yes, these are all great neutrals, because they work with pretty much any other colour. As such, they're probably also the colours you are prepared to spend more money on. Think about it – would you rather spend a greater amount on a black or grey winter coat than a trendy red one?

Think of an item you may have seen or purchased and recall the terms used to describe the colour. Brands come up with all sorts of ambiguous words to describe a colour. Is it brown or burgundy? No, it's grape. Is it green or grey? No, it's olive. Is it orange or brown? No, it's nutmeg. These colours are what I mean by alternative neutrals. Surprisingly (and pleasingly) they will work just as hard for you, be just as versatile, will work harmoniously with your traditional neutrals and, dare I say it, may even be just a little more stylish.

Let's use olive as a neutral and show it alongside navy and black in the same outfit to test my theory. In the first set we have lilac as our pop colour and set it against olive, then navy. In the second set we have red as our pop colour and set it against olive, then black.

Can you see that olive green can indeed be a neutral? And when paired with other combinations, it's possibly more interesting than navy or black?

If you want to lean into looking more creative and unique, take a look at your wardrobe and start to create some new outfits based around a non-traditional neutral. Although 'less obvious' neutrals, they will already be in your wardrobe if they are colours you love. One of my favourites is olive green, but yours might be peach, caramel, soft blue, burgundy or chocolate brown. To start, you may only have one or two pieces in this 'new' neutral and that's okay. Let's start there! Working this colour into your outfits doesn't mean having to throw out your existing neutrals – it's just an opportunity to broaden your choices and experiment with colour combinations to enhance and diversify your personal style. Once you discover a new neutral that works for you, shop with this colour in mind. Centring your wardrobe around a more unusual hue will help to develop your own signature, stylish look.

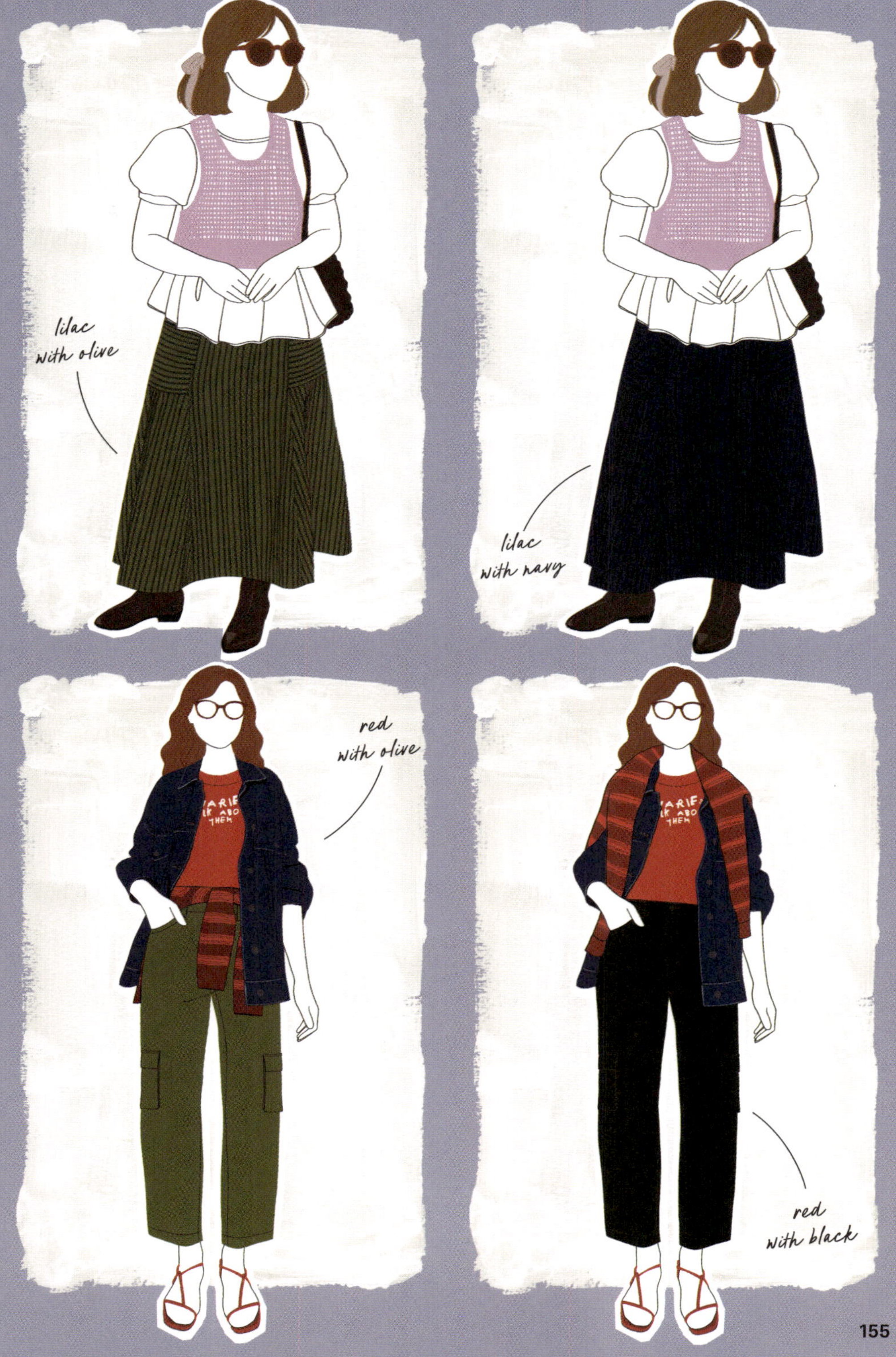

lilac
with olive
lilac
with navy
red
with olive
red
with black

What colours work for you?

My approach to colours aligns with my approach to styling in general: there are no rules; wear what makes you feel good!

Every now and then the idea of having a 'set' of colours that suits you best pops up. As with Bev, this is likely to change for many reasons. Just like everyone's skin tone is different, so too will be everyone's version of grey hair. Some will be salt and pepper, others silver and others a grey blonde, or even white. There is no 'one size fits all', which is why being aware of and adapting to change is the best way to ensure you can always feel your best. It's also why the simple activity at the beginning of this chapter is worth revisiting over time. When you experience a significant change – hair colour, even hair length – do the activity again and experiment with some new colours too. See how you feel. Do some shades work better now than others? Do you need to adjust your make-up?

You can also apply this theory to the changes of season. Sometimes the colours we like to wear and feel our best in can change depending on the weather. You might tan really easily in summer and therefore feel great wearing pastels more so than in winter. Pastels might also provide you with a feeling you associate with warmer weather (or even holidays), and therefore give you a sense of happiness, calm or joy when you wear them. In winter you might be drawn to colours like charcoal, burgundy and navy because they instil a sense of comfort and warmth.

Here's something to think about. Your favourite colour might be red but what would happen if the shade of red that you've been told is your 'best red' is not easily found in the brands you like to shop from? They might sell *a* red but it's not quite the 'right' red for you, according to your assigned colour chart. What if you happen to find your 'perfect red jumper' while searching online but it's from a designer label that is well out of your budget. Do you spend money you cannot afford to simply own the perfect red jumper? I would argue that, no, you should not. I would suggest you keep an open mind and instead try on various shades of red from brands within your budget and assess how you feel in those.

Through trial and error, you'll soon discover that some reds feel intuitively 'better' than others. Perhaps some reds will simply feel more 'you' than others. Do they have to be the 'perfect red'? No. Might they elicit the same happy, positive feelings as wearing your 'perfect red'? Yes. Rather than limiting your choices, you're extending them simply by being open to more possibilities. Equally, it's important to think about what item you are considering. Is it a red jumper or a red handbag? If the latter, I'd say, 'Does it *really* matter if it's your perfect red?'

Another scenario might be that you finally find a bright pink coat after years of hunting for one. It ticks all your boxes in terms of length, form, functionality and price point but you consult your colour guide only to discover the coat is not your 'best pink'. What do you do? Not try the coat on and keep looking for another five years? When we're told that we can only wear particular shades of any colour, we miss out on buying or wearing items that we may truly love and feel great in.

Think outside the box

I encourage you to think outside the box when considering your wardrobe and style palette, including your so-called neutrals. Don't be afraid to update your wardrobe over the seasons – whether to lean into a trend or update your collection to suit your current mood and lifestyle. As we learnt from Indi and Steph in Chapter 3, colour can be the difference between a core and a charisma purchase and will help you express your style personality. Colour is a magic wand in your personal styling toolkit and soon you'll learn how to rely on it when it comes to smart packing. And your colour choice doesn't always have to be bold – if you don't want to make a big commitment, using make-up and accessories can be an ideal way to add some subtle colour to your look and to refresh your style.

Colour is a *magic wand* in your personal styling toolkit.

Three

Endless Inspiration

Your life will *evolve*,
and with that,
    your wardrobe
will too.

12. SHOP LIKE A PRO

I'm a personal shopper, so it's my job to be good at shopping for clothes. If I could recall the number of times a client has said, 'There's no way I could have bought all those pieces in two or three hours on my own!' I'd probably have enough words for another book.

I understand, though, that shopping is not something everyone finds joy in. For many people buying clothes can be tedious, stressful, frustrating and even depressing. It can be overwhelming for starters. Online, in store, second-hand, handmade – the choices are endless. Shopping for clothes is literally at our fingertips, with online fashion becoming more and more popular and social media platforms now selling straight from our feeds. And while we've come a long way in terms of the accessibility of a variety of brands and price points, ethical and sustainable choices and size inclusivity, we've got a way to go.

Sometimes having too much to choose from makes it more challenging to shop with intent and purpose. Throw in all the factors already covered – our wardrobe purpose, style personality, body shape, colours, age, budget . . . and it's a lot! So, let me give you a roadmap for shopping just like I do: with a plan and with a purpose.

Advance planning

When we walk into a clothing store without a gameplan, that's when things can go awry – just like going to the supermarket without a list or when we're hungry. We can be influenced by what others say, such as sales assistants and our friends, and go home having spent way too much money on something we don't even really like that much. When we shop without a plan, we're also more likely to get sidetracked by something we don't need, or even truly want but, damn, it looks amazing in the moment. And when we go shopping without enough time, we make impulsive decisions. Similarly, if we've had a crap day or week, and we're wanting that dopamine hit to make us feel better, we may buy something so outrageously out of our budget that we return it the next week.

If we don't get clear on what we're shopping for, we often end up buying the same item we already have several of hanging in our wardrobes. Are you starting to see the importance of shopping with intention and with purpose? So here are the things I do *before* I set out on a shopping expedition.

Create a shopping list

When I shop with a client, we don't just browse the stores for a few hours, waiting for things to 'jump out' at us. We shop with a plan – a shopping list! It's so simple but it works. The list is what we use to stay on track, to maintain our focus and to know exactly what we're looking for in any shop we're in – including online! Sure, you might get led astray here and there but if you can try to stick to what's on the list and avoid things that aren't on it, you're off to a great start.

This predetermined list is crucial in ensuring we don't overspend, overbuy or waste time trying on things that we don't need. You too should shop with a list. Think about what it is that you really want and write it down. Take the time to assess what's in your wardrobe and write down what you'd like to add that will work with your existing pieces – and enhance them.

Using your wardrobe purpose, style personality and Three Cs to assess your wardrobe gaps will help keep you on track and focused on what your wardrobe needs and what you'll wear 80 per cent of the time. Looking back at your saved folder or Pinterest board of style inspiration will also help with this and give you ideas for useful items to shop for.

Set a budget

When I work with clients, knowing their budget is imperative. This will determine what stores we shop in, because without it, how am I to know if they want to spend $300 on a winter coat or $3000? So, as part of your shopping list, assign a budget to each item.

I would argue knowing and sticking to your budget during sale time is even more important. It's so easy to get sucked in by a good sale but just because something is cheaper than usual doesn't mean it's a good buy, especially if it's still out of your budget! It's just not worth it. Don't let the allure of the sale or the feeling of 'missing out' impact your decision-making.

Where sales *are* good is if a sale item is something you've been coveting. For example, if you've had your eye on a piece all season, saved it in your style inspiration folder and thought about whether it aligns with your style personality and serves your wardrobe purpose, now might be the time to buy!

What I'm really talking about is impulse shopping. We've all done it but having a list that you've really thought through will help avoid bringing home something simply because it's on sale. My advice? Keep walking (or scrolling) 99 per cent of the time.

Know your brands

We want shopping for clothes to be fun, joyful and successful, so it's important to not set yourself up for failure. Knowing a brand's size range and price point before you enter a store is crucial to keeping your shopping experience positive. Because I'm a personal shopper, it's my job to do this for my clients.

Doing some homework online before you shop will help keep you on track and maximise your time. Once you've determined what stores cater for your size range and budget, you can start to narrow in on what specific items you plan to look at or try on.

For example, if a new trench coat is on your shopping list and your budget is around $300, you want to have a few options to go and try on, knowing which stores have trench coats in your price range. If you've already determined where some items on your shopping list are available within your budget, you can organise your shopping trip to make it more seamless. You might simply bookmark the items in your internet browser, keep screenshots or paste the URLs into your notes for quick reference.

Many stores also now have a 'find in store' function on their websites. This is a fabulous tool I use regularly to ensure the size I want to try is available – again, setting myself up for shopping success, not failure.

I also like to use a website's 'wishlist' function to keep track of items I like from one store. By creating a profile with the brand (which you may already have if it's a favourite), you can add items to your wishlist and sometimes set alerts if they go on sale. Wishlists are also really great 'placeholders' for items you like but don't necessarily need. I've often saved something to a wishlist thinking I'll go back the next day to purchase, only to completely forget about it! It's amazing how giving yourself a little bit of time to think about something often leaves you not thinking about it at all.

Dana goes shopping

Dana, like many others, had put on weight during the pandemic and needed some new clothes when she returned to in-person work. She was very clear about wanting to maintain the image she had always portrayed in the workplace – approachable, professional, modern – and was quick to recall all her old favourite stores she used to shop in to achieve this look.

Dana had already provided me with the usual information I get from clients before working with them, including her size, shopping list and budget, so I'd already earmarked items I wanted to show her and stores I wanted to take her to that matched these criteria.

After our initial coffee and chat to confirm the desired outcomes for the session, it was obvious Dana was unsure about her actual current size because she hadn't been shopping for some time. Off we went into our first store, a brand Dana had never shopped in before but which I knew would work for her shape, size and style. We browsed and I selected pieces in a range of sizes (it's always worth taking at least two sizes of the same item to try on), and we headed to the fitting room.

Dana emerged wearing outfit number one. She looked great. She felt great. Everything fitted her perfectly. The joy and delight on Dana's face were obvious, as well as a sense of relief. Dana hadn't felt confident about maintaining her old style at her new size. However, because I ensured that the first thing I asked her to try on fit well, her self-confidence was restored and her sense of style reinstated. This meant that the rest of the shopping session went swimmingly because Dana was now feeling positive about shopping, empowered in her choices and more self-assured in herself and her personal style.

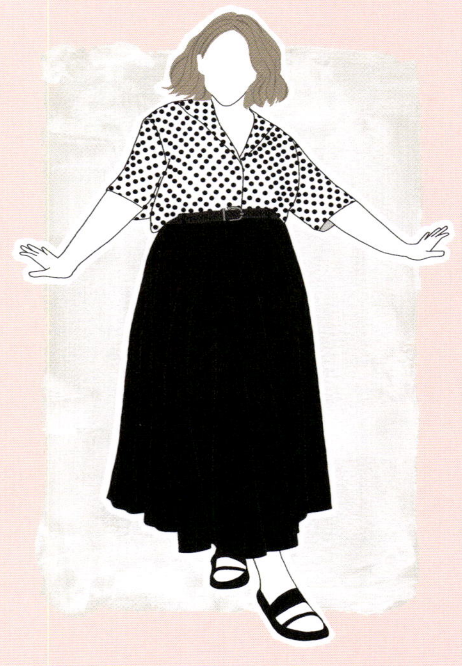

On the day

You've set aside the time to go shopping, you have your plan and budget ready. Now what? Let me take you through some of my most important tips for a successful shopping trip that I use with my clients.

Allow yourself time

How often have you raced into the shops on your lunchbreak, before the school pick-up or on the day of an event only to purchase something you didn't really like because it was the 'best you could find'? When we're rushed, we make hasty decisions. It's important to give yourself enough time to shop properly: time to browse, time to try on different sizes, time to think, consider, take photos and contemplate.

Remember, it's okay to try something on in a store and walk out empty handed. It's okay to say to the sales assistant, 'Thanks, I just need to think about it.' Why do we find that so hard to do? I believe that we feel a sense of obligation in these situations – for taking up someone's time (even though that's their job!) – and so we feel we owe it to them to purchase. Or perhaps we feel like we're being judged that we can't afford whatever we just tried on, and so we want to prove them wrong.

When you shop with intention and plenty of time, you'll be able to confidently tell the sales assistant that you're going to think about it and leave a store empty handed rather than with a bag of clothes you aren't sure about. Or, if you're shopping online, you'll be able to leave your cart overnight so that you can come back to it in the morning with a fresh perspective, or after you've had time to compare measurements or look for more budget-friendly alternatives.

Giving myself time to think about adding a new item of clothing into my wardrobe has been one of the best strategies I've employed to help me be a better shopper. Allowing yourself time also applies when you do make a purchase. Sometimes we need to take something home to try on in order to assess it with more objectivity. Nothing beats trying a new piece on with your existing favourites to see if it's going to work, and sometimes you need to be in your own space, with your own mirror and the lighting you're used to, to really tell if you like something.

Now that we're shopping online more than ever, I believe it's even more important to take the time to try things on, create a few new looks and take some photos to decide if you want to keep them or return them. You're allowed to change your mind. In most cases you can return an item for a refund if it's not quite right – but do check the return policy before purchasing! And if you do decide to return something, do it as soon as you can. Some policies have small windows for refunds, and when you miss them it's an unnecessary cost to bear.

Make it fun

Clothes shopping can release dopamine, our body's natural feel-good chemicals. The anticipation of finding something new and desirable can trigger the brain's reward system, giving us a rush even before the actual purchase. We all know that feeling of pure joy when we score something on sale that we've been coveting, nab the last item in our size or simply buy something that we'd dreamed of owning. Successfully finding and purchasing an item that fits well and looks good can create a sense of accomplishment and satisfaction. And let's not forget that new clothes allow us to express our personal style and identity. When we get it right, this helps to enhance our self-esteem and overall wellbeing, which also contributes to us feeling good.

However, there's another factor that plays into the release of these feel-good chemicals when it comes to shopping – novelty and variety. The constant release of new fashion trends, not to mention seasonal collections, continues to stimulate the brain's pleasure centres. It's non-stop! Be careful that this doesn't lead to negative consequences, such as financial stress or compulsive buying behaviour. The allure of new clothes is exciting but not to the detriment of one's health, self-esteem or financial situation.

Shop on your own

You have the knowledge, you know your style and your wardrobe, and hopefully you've now got an increased sense of confidence to shop with intention. With your tools at hand (i.e. this book!), you're going to be your own personal shopper! Whenever you can, shop on your own, including without your children, if possible, so you can truly focus on yourself. (I acknowledge this may be more difficult if you have young children.)

When we shop with others, as well intended as they may be, we are often steered off course. We can be swayed by their opinions rather than listening to our own, and we let their tastes, values and bias influence ours. We may feel bad for disagreeing with them and may sometimes even feel bullied into buying something.

Susan goes shopping

Susan's husband, Geoff, organised a personal shopping session for Susan for their twenty-year wedding anniversary, and she was so excited; she'd never done anything like this before. She was a confident, professional woman who led a large team in corporate finance. Her style was simple, somewhat conservative and a little dated.

Susan brought Geoff along for the session or, should I say, Geoff brought Susan. After our initial chat over a cup of coffee, it was clear that Susan was keen to try some new things, explore some new brands and update her look. We headed off to our first store and I started selecting pieces for her. As I always do, I asked, 'What do you think of this?' Susan looked at the item, then Geoff, then me. She was unsure but eager to try. 'I'm in your hands, Sally!' she said.

As we made our way to the changing room, arms spilling with lots of new pieces and combinations to try, Susan's eagerness was obvious. I hung up all the items in categories and suggested she try on a pair of jeans with a blouse, and I'd bring her some shoes to complete the look. Geoff took a seat just outside.

Susan emerged looking absolutely incredible, a huge smile on her face. I asked if it was okay for me to do some adjustments, and then tucked in her top, pulled up the sleeves a touch, shortened the jeans to remove the excess fabric and gave her the shoes to put on.

Susan looked in the mirror. 'Wow! I would never have tried these jeans on myself. My legs look so much longer,' she said.

I asked, 'So how do you feel with the top tucked in to the jeans?'

'I thought it was going to show off my stomach,' she said, 'but I can see that it's doing the opposite. And this colour – I would never have chosen it, but I really like it.'

Susan walked out to show Geoff, feeling great about herself. She was seeing herself

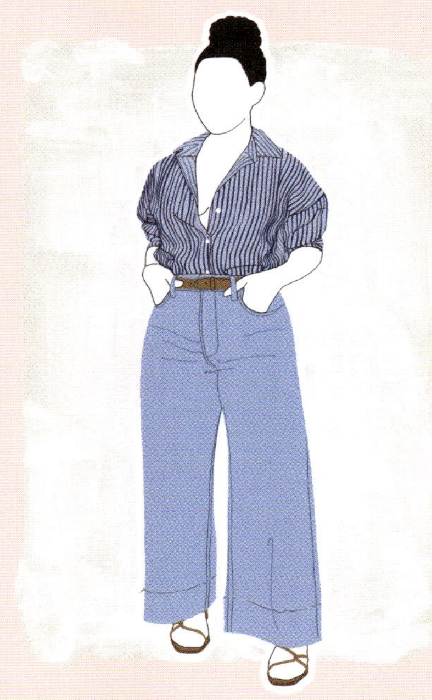

differently, and she liked it very much. With her eyes full of delight, her gaze met Geoff's. And in that moment, everything changed. Without saying a word it was clear that Geoff didn't approve of Susan's new look. He didn't want her to change or 'show off her figure'. He'd organised the session for her thinking it would be a bit of fun and hadn't expected such a transformation. The light in Susan's eyes immediately diminished. Her confidence was suddenly shattered. It was instant. And it was frustrating and saddening to watch.

This is a scenario I've faced with clients from time to time when a significant other – be it sister, son, daughter, mother, wife, friend – comes along but rather than being there for moral support they become the antagonist.

I want you to keep this in mind the next time you go shopping with someone else, or ask someone their opinion on how you look, because the only person who can truly provide honest, objective feedback is yourself.

What to wear (and what not to wear)

Another thing you can do to set yourself up for success when you shop is to wear something you feel really good in. Get dressed to go shopping! Put on something that makes you feel confident, that you really love and that reflects your style personality.

Good underwear

First things first: underwear. I have always advised my clients to wear a 'good set of nude knickers and bra' to come shopping with me. What do I mean by good? Well, a bra that is supportive, fits well and is not a sports bra. Same goes for knickers. If you're planning to shop for occasion wear, jeans, summer dresses – most things really – you want underwear that is supportive and will allow whatever you're trying on to be the star of the show, so ideally something seamless or minimal. If you would typically wear shapewear of any sort under the clothing you are shopping for, bring it along to put on if you don't want to wear it all day. Similarly, if you're planning to shop for clothing that will require a strapless bra, take one with you.

The right shoes

Shoes matter too. Wear something comfy if you're going to be walking around a lot but if you want to wear heels with whatever you're shopping for, bring a pair of heels with you. Many women struggle to imagine how something will look with the 'right' shoe. If you're setting out to buy a new pair of full-length pants, wear or bring along a pair of shoes you're most likely to wear with them. We can no longer rely on stores to have a 'try-on' pair of shoes for us to use due to health and safety reasons, so we need to take these matters into our own hands – or should I say feet!

Easy clothing

You also want to choose clothing that is easy to take on and off, including your shoes, so I would recommend not wearing sneakers. Unlacing them and lacing them up again is very time consuming and will drive you insane, so choose something you can easily slip on and off, like a ballet flat, slide, slip-on boot or loafer.

For the same reasons, I recommend that you avoid wearing anything with too many buttons. Tops and bottoms that you can easily fling off and on again are ideal, rather than a button-up shirt, a blouse or a dress with fiddly buttons.

You should also consider what you're shopping for. For example, if you're shopping for a new jacket or coat, and you would typically wear a jacket or coat with jeans or pants, don't wear a dress or skirt. If you're shopping for a new pair of jeans, it will be easier if you're wearing a top and bottom instead of a dress so that you can assess them with a more accurate eye (rather than with your dress held up around your waist!).

Do your hair and make-up

While we're talking about how you look on the outside, don't dismiss how you're feeling on the inside. Shopping can be demoralising at the best of times, so if you're not feeling your best, choose another time. Try to go shopping when you are in a good frame of mind, have the energy to try things on and are feeling confident in yourself.

Along with choosing an outfit to look and feel your best, don't forget about your hair and make-up. If you usually wear make-up, wear it to go shopping. You're going to be standing in front of a mirror (undoubtedly under terrible lighting!) assessing yourself and how you look, so why not feel your best?

If you usually wear your hair down, then wear your hair down. You'll be amazed at how seeing your hair against a colour affects your decision-making or even how a neckline frames your face. Similarly, if you usually wear your hair up, that's how you should wear it to go shopping. You want the shopping experience to reflect your real life as much as possible.

Clothes shopping can release dopamine, our body's *natural feel-good* chemical.

Get out there and shop (with intention)!

If you've got this far into the book, I hope you're starting to see the connection between knowing your true sense of style and wardrobe purpose and being an intentional and successful shopper. It all comes full circle, and it's a win-win all round.

These ideas and suggestions are not about placing arbitrary restrictions on your spending habits or to thwart your love of clothing and fashion. They're designed to give you the power to wear and buy clothing that presents the person you want to be.

So, the next time you go to buy something I want you to:

STOP: Pause before purchasing!

THINK: Think about how it's going to work with your wardrobe and fit into your lifestyle. Will it serve a purpose 80 per cent of the time and align with your style personality?

WAIT: Wait a day before purchasing. If you wake up the next morning and can't stop thinking about it, and it's still available in your size, then it's meant to be.

ASSESS: Just because you couldn't stop thinking about it and you bought it, doesn't mean it's always right. Take the time to assess whether it's a keep or return (and do so as soon as you can).

No matter what you're shopping for, when you plan ahead, dress for success and bring your well thought out list, your shopping trip will be far more productive, time efficient and successful.

13. ORGANISE YOUR WARDROBE

An organised wardrobe is a game changer, from helping us to get dressed more quickly to knowing what's missing from our wardrobes. It's also integral to facilitating everything we've discussed so far.

You may already have a system and if it's working for you, you don't have to change it. But working with thousands of wardrobes over the years has given me some pretty good insights into how a wardrobe can be made most efficient.

The advice in this chapter will apply to you regardless of your personal style, the size of your wardrobe, your lifestyle and your budget. It's also relevant no matter what your newly identified wardrobe purpose, style personality and Three Cs might be.

Categorise your clothes

Whatever your wardrobe size or layout, I advise categorising your clothes. That means bringing like-for-like items together into the one space. Let's look at how this works in retail and you'll see how it affects our response to our clothes.

When we go shopping in a large department store, each brand/designer is allocated their own space (called a 'concession') in which to feature a capsule selection of items on a few racks. The items are not typically displayed in any particular order, and one concession may be set up completely differently to the next. When we shop in such stores, we often spend quite some time sifting through the racks in search of what we like. There seems to be no rhyme or reason as to how the store is merchandised. While brands may be grouped in loose connection with each other (by price/age/gender), each collection is unique to that brand and their current collection. And that's what draws us to department stores: the variety, the choice! Oh, the choice!

Sometimes we want to browse, and department stores are great for that, with so many designers on one floor. But how many times have you shopped in a department store and felt overwhelmed, confused and given up? How many times have you struggled to find what you're looking for because it's not obvious where to find it, and left feeling deflated and frustrated?

Now, let's compare the department store experience to a single-brand store like Uniqlo. Uniqlo merchandise every single item of clothing into categories. So, when you walk into a store, you'll find every category of an item in one place. For example, I go to Uniqlo every winter for a cashmere jumper in a new colour. When I walk into the store, I go straight to the spot where all the cashmere jumpers are located, take a look, choose the colour I like, and done. No browsing aimlessly trying to locate what I'm there to buy, no wasting precious time, and no getting sidetracked by things I don't need.

This is how your wardrobe should work for you too. Everything in categories, side by side, where you can see them and, most importantly, locate them. There are many advantages of this method of organisation.

Know where everything is

When your wardrobe is organised by category, and you need a long-sleeve button-down shirt, they're all there hanging side by side. Perhaps you want a silk version to dress up your jeans, and that will be sitting just next to the cotton ones. If you want a cashmere jumper to throw casually over your shoulders, they're all folded neatly in a drawer. Bang, bang, bang. You'll spend almost no time searching for what you're looking for. How many times have you rustled through your wardrobe looking for a particular pair of black pants? Whether you have two pairs or twenty, you'll find them with ease when they're all hanging together.

See outfits in your wardrobe before trying them on

When your wardrobe is organised, you'll find it easier to identify what you want to wear. You will seamlessly scan your wardrobe and see items that you can build an outfit from. This can help to speed up your everyday decision-making process, because you'll start to visualise your ensemble before you even try it on. This is true even when you're not standing in front of your wardrobe! The next time you're out shopping and thinking to yourself, 'What could I wear this with?', you'll be able to picture your wardrobe and know exactly the answer.

Identify what you've got a lot of and what's missing

Another advantage of wardrobe categorisation is that it will become obvious what your wardrobe is both heaving with and lacking in. When you can see those twenty pairs of black pants all hanging together, you'll be more likely to ask yourself, 'Do I really need another pair?' When you go to choose a jacket for a night out with friends and only have a hiking fleece on hand, you'll know you're missing outerwear options. Knowing what your wardrobe is lacking can help you be a more considered shopper. Unless an item is looking tired or feels dated and you're ready to part with it, can you make do with the options you already have? This method will also help you to confirm your style personality, because I guarantee that the items in your wardrobe that you have multiples of are indeed core pieces that define your personal style.

Get dressed with greater ease and purpose

Organising your wardrobe in this way will help you get dressed with greater efficiency and give you the most effective use of your wardrobe. When you can see everything, you're much more likely to fully utilise your wardrobe, mixing the old with the new. When we don't store similar pieces together, we often end up wearing the things we've purchased most recently on high rotation simply because we can see them. But when we are diligent about maintaining an organised wardrobe, we might just choose a different piece the next time for a totally new experience!

An organised
wardrobe is a
game changer.

Make the most of your wardrobe storage

Regardless of your wardrobe size, there are certain clothing items that I recommend hanging and certain things I recommend folding and storing on shelves or in drawers. Jackets, coats, silk shirts, blouses, dresses, skirts and trousers are all best on hangers for a variety of reasons, if you have the space, whereas things like jumpers are better suited to being folded.

The more of your wardrobe you can hang, the easier it is to see it. The items you choose to hang should generally be your core and charisma modules as you want these to be easily accessible. You want to look after and appreciate these pieces (they're probably the ones you've spent the most money on), so they deserve to be well treated. Hanging them helps to maintain their shape and means they're less likely to need an iron or steam when you want to wear them.

Jackets and coats

A coathanger mimics the human shoulder line, which means it's a practical and obvious tool for hanging jackets and coats. A good, strong coathanger will keep the shoulders of your coats in good shape (literally). Coats and jackets are also rather tricky to fold – if you've travelled with one, you'll know how hard they are to wrangle into your suitcase. Hanging them is so much easier *and* will take up less space.

Dresses

You likely have dresses in your wardrobe of different lengths and fabrics. Hang them all but group them in categories, with formal dresses together, then strappy summer dresses, work dresses and so on, side by side. There might be the occasional t-shirt dress that you prefer to fold and tuck away in a drawer with your t-shirts but, for the most part, dresses are best stored on hangers. Ideally, hang your dresses and long coats where they have room to fall all the way to the floor, to limit creasing. Otherwise, use a second hanger to lift the length off the floor. Keep all your longer items hanging to one side of your wardrobe for maximum space, drape and visibility.

Shirts and blouses

Shirts and blouses, be they cotton, silk or synthetic, will fall and drape better on a hanger, and it helps them avoid getting creased, so you can take them straight out of your wardrobe and wear them.

Skirts and trousers

Like other 'hanger-worthy' items, skirts and trousers prefer to hang and fall, just like they do on our bodies, particularly those styles that are longer and have more fabric, such as a midi-length pleated skirt or a wide-leg full-length trouser.

For skirts and tailored trousers, the best hangers are the ones where you can clip them either side of the waistband. If you're short on space, some pants or trousers will happily work folded over a regular coathanger – such as a drill cotton cargo pant, a casual linen pant or a weekend jogger. My general rule of thumb here comes down to fabric – the sturdier the fabric, the more likely you can store it folded on a hanger or folded in a drawer.

Ideally, limit the number of skirts or trousers on each hanger to a maximum of two.

Remember, you're trying to maximise how much of your wardrobe you can see and access easily. When we have multiple items on one hanger, we can no longer see what's there and might forget our favourite items because they're hiding between two other pairs of pants or skirts we don't wear as much. They can also get quite heavy!

Knitwear

Have you ever reached for your favourite woollen jumper only to put it on and realise the coathanger has left an annoying bump on each shoulder? This is my number one reason for *not* hanging my knitwear. The finer and more delicate the knit (such as merino and cashmere), the more likely a coathanger will leave marks. It can also stretch. The heavier the knit and the wider the gauge, the more likely it will lose its shape on a hanger.

Also, some knitwear is really chunky. Those delicious cosy jumpers and cardigans that feel like they're giving you a big hug when you wear them can take up a lot of space hanging in your wardrobe. Why do you think puffer jackets are designed to roll and pack away in the summer months? I prefer to fold knitwear and store it in a drawer or on a shelf. Again, keep similar items together in one spot where you can see and access them.

If you don't have any drawers or shelves or are simply hellbent on hanging your fine knitwear, ensure your coathangers have some padding that will keep the shoulders of your knits from stretching.

Jeans

How many pairs of jeans you own will affect where and how you store them. If you're a big denim lover like me, the most space-efficient way to store them is folded and stacked in piles (and piles!) on top of each other, since they're quite bulky and will take up a lot of space hanging in your wardrobe. Also, jeans don't crease as easily as cotton, wool or silk pants, so they can be folded. They will still be easily accessible, especially if you have them folded on a shelf rather than in a drawer. If, on the other hand, you only own a few pairs, then you might decide to hang them alongside your other pants.

T-shirts

You might be sensing by now that the dressier pieces in your wardrobe deserve to be hung, whereas the more casual ones can be relegated to a shelf or drawer. Case in point, the t-shirt. While they might be a core piece in your wardrobe, they don't really need to be displayed on a hanger and can be neatly folded and stored in a drawer or stacked on a shelf.

Shoes

There are two camps of people when it comes to shoe storage: those who keep the boxes when they buy new shoes and those who don't. I personally like to keep my shoes in their original boxes because it allows me to keep them organised, takes up less space and keeps them dust free. If you're someone who has a delightfully generous walk-in wardrobe with dedicated shoe shelves, lucky you! Or you might have a compact space yet enough built-in drawers for shoes – also, lucky you! Or perhaps you're someone who stores their shoes in clear boxes – if that works for you, stick to it.

If you don't have any of the above options for shoes, I have a few suggestions. First, keep only the shoes you wear on high rotation (at any given time of the year) placed on the floor of your wardrobe. The rest can be stored away in storage boxes elsewhere. Depending on the size of your wardrobe (and general storage space in your home) these boxes or tubs could be in your wardrobe, under your bed or in another cupboard. The important thing is to keep this tub somewhere that is easy to access and keep 'refreshing' it as the seasons (and your wardrobe) change.

An example of this is sandal season versus boot season. In the depths of winter, you can safely put away your strappy sandals (unless you, like me, have declassified them!) and have only your boots or other enclosed shoes on display. Come summer, simply switch them over. Second, now that you've got a more organised closet space, perhaps there is a spare drawer, shelf or compartment where you can neatly store some of your shoes? Again, if space is tight, choose the shoes you wear most frequently to be easily accessible, and the rest can be stored away.

The tools I recommend

I've long been of the opinion that regardless of how much money you spend, you should always look after and care for your clothing. A $15 white cotton shirt from Kmart that is clean and freshly ironed will always look better than a $1500 stained, unironed one! Likewise, the inexpensive polyester blouse that you send to the drycleaner because you love the colour so much and every time you wear it, it feels brand new. For this reason, the tools you have at your disposal for storing your clothes affect how long your clothes last and how you feel when you approach your wardrobe.

Coathangers

It might sound irrelevant but the hangers you choose are quite crucial in wardrobe organisation. I have visited many homes and seen all sorts of wardrobes, and the thing that always shocks me is when someone has a beautiful wardrobe full of designer clothes that are methodically organised, with built-in shoe and bag racks and . . . wire coathangers!

Regardless of our budgets, we can all display our clothing in a way that looks beautiful, feels inviting and works efficiently simply by organising them and displaying them in a particular way. Matching coathangers are our secret weapon because they look appealing and more luxe. You don't have to throw out all your coathangers to achieve this today. Buy five at a time, slowly weeding out all the flimsy wire ones you got from the drycleaners and bringing in sleek but sturdy replacements. These are my favourites:

Wooden hangers – for heavy coats and jackets

Wooden hangers are perfect because they support both the structure and weight of jackets and coats, maintaining a garment's shoulder line.

Flocked hangers – for dresses, blazers and tops

Flocked hangers look great! Whatever the colour (I like to keep consistent) these hangers will not only leave your closet looking neat, organised and 'boutique'-like, but also serve a practical purpose. Being narrow, they don't take up too much space, and the velvet coating means your clothing won't slip off.

Hangers with clips – for skirts and trousers

Hangers with clips have lots of benefits. First, it means the garments hang lengthways, just like they do in a shop, meaning no annoying creases (the ones you get from folding skirts and trousers over a hanger). Second, a vertically hanging skirt or trouser takes up less space. And third, a hanging garment is much easier to see and access when on clips than folded over a regular coathanger.

And why no wire coathangers? Because they don't keep your clothing 'in shape'. A wire hanger won't support the shoulders of your blazer, protect the fabric of your silk blouse or bear the weight of your chunky cable knit sweater. They may take up less space but wire hangers look disposable and because they easily bend out of shape, they also look messy and cheap. Remember, our wardrobes are where we house the clothes we buy to reflect the person we want to be. Respecting our clothes by being considerate of their placement, storage and condition impacts how we feel when we wear them.

Hanging hooks

I love using hooks to hang things on and I use them inside my closet, on the back of doors – anywhere there's a space to hang something. You can use them to start building your outfits, to help you visualise how items might work together. They're a great way to display what you're planning to wear the next day.

They can also be a handy storage tool when you don't have a lot of wardrobe space. Those big hooks that go over doors can go on the back of your bedroom door so you can hang up a couple of coats. Multiple hooks on the inside of a wardrobe door or on a wall are great for hanging accessories like necklaces or scarves. They don't take up much room but the efficiency of having these everyday items hanging and visible means you're more likely to reach for them.

A full-length mirror

When you go shopping, you take items to the fitting room and try them on with the full-length mirror to determine if you like the look of them. You might turn sideways, spin around to assess the rear view or check the length of the pants with the shoes you're wearing. And you should do exactly the same thing in your own home.

A mirror is a non-negotiable, in my opinion. It's an essential tool for building outfits (as discussed in Chapter 8) and will allow you to assess your outfit and make changes, tweaks and adjustments when getting dressed. When you can see yourself from head to toe, you can see how the proportions of your outfit work, or not.

When you can only see yourself from the waist up in your bathroom or dresser mirror, the only part of your outfit you're objectively assessing is your top half. And no, standing on your toilet so you can see yourself from head to toe does not count as having a full-length mirror! (True story . . . and I've heard it more than once!) The best place for a full-length mirror is where you get dressed, or as close to it as possible, so in your bedroom or in your wardrobe is ideal.

Think of a full-length mirror as your objective stylist. I appreciate that for some people, looking in mirrors is not an easy or enjoyable task. But hopefully by this point in the book, you're already starting to feel more confident and empowered regarding your personal style and therefore more open and willing to look at yourself. A mirror is not a tool for being critical or judgemental of yourself, it's a tool to help you explore the possibilities within your wardrobe, to play, to experiment, to have fun. It's what allows you to see how fabulous you look, to see the person looking back at you and smile, because, damn, you look good!

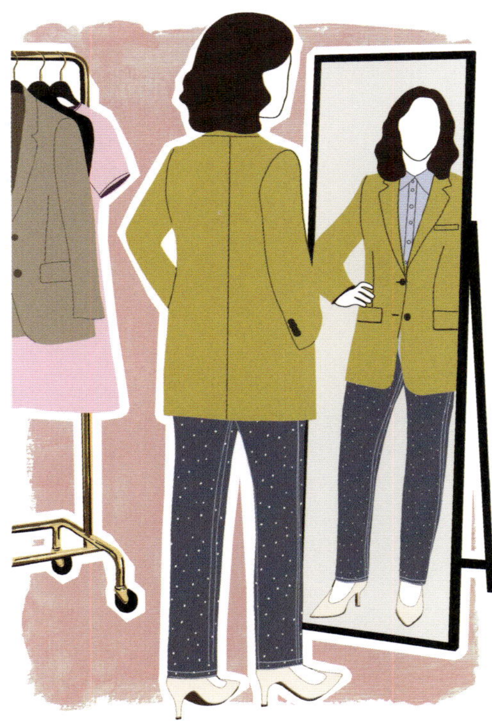

What if I have a small wardrobe space?

At this point, you might very well be wondering how you can achieve the above outcomes in a tight space. The principles are still the same and, I would argue, even more important.

First, prioritise what items should be hung – ideally your jackets, coats, shirts, blouses, dresses, skirts and trousers. Of these, start by prioritising the ones that are part of your core.

These deserve prime hanging space in your wardrobe. In terms of the rest, could you pack away a few items that you know you won't be wearing this season? For example, if it's summer, perhaps your core winter pieces could be packed away or vice versa.

Can other items make do on a shelf or in a drawer? For example, if I had a silk dress that I wore at least once a week to work, then that would take priority in my wardrobe because I don't want to iron it every time I wear it, whereas a knitted long-sleeve dress that I only wear in the depths of winter can remain folded in a drawer with my jumpers until the seasons change.

If there are 'out of season' items you can store, you might be able to put them in large plastic tubs under your bed. They're still fairly easy to access if you need them. When space is limited, tools like hooks are also a great way to instantly create more hanging space, as mentioned previously.

Worth the effort

Ultimately, it is worth spending some time, energy and money in organising your wardrobe, as categorising and taking care of your clothes will help you build outfits more easily and you'll feel less frustrated when you can wear clothes straight off the hanger or drawer. Your beautifully organised wardrobe doesn't have to happen overnight. Start working on your closet section by section, hanger by hanger. And when you're done, I promise you that the wardrobe looking back at you will be just as easy to 'shop from' as your local Uniqlo store.

14. KEEP YOUR WARDROBE FRESH

Hopefully by now you're realising that personal style has nothing to do with where you shop, how much you spend or what size you are. But something that can impact your personal style – and applies to everyone – is how you care for your clothes. I'm all about clothing longevity, whether something is an investment or a cheap and cheerful purchase. Some of these things you might already do but I hope some are new ideas that will help you extend the life of your favourite pieces.

There are a number of 'hacks' that I've been employing for years without really thinking too much about them, and they're all things that make my life easier and my wardrobe more wearable. These tips might sound like such simple things (and they are) but they will change your life!

Handle your clothes with care

Caring for your clothes is much more than just putting your delicates in the washing machine on a gentle cycle or not putting your jeans in the dryer. Here are my favourite tips.

Get out the scissors

When you buy a new jacket or coat (and sometimes skirts), check for stitching on the rear vent. A vent is the single (sometimes double) opening on the back of a garment that is sewn shut during manufacturing. The purpose of this stitching is to keep the vent in place while it's being transported, stored, hung and tried on but it's not designed to stay on the garment once purchased. Removing it will allow more flexible movement in the garment, which is a very good thing, so snip it off. I've lost count of the number of people I've seen in public (including wedding parties, in business meetings, on the TV and even my own staff members!) with their vent stitching still intact. It's such a simple and easy thing to do but unfortunately, even when you buy a jacket in store, the salesperson will rarely advise you to do it. While you've got out the scissors, here are a few other annoying things you can chop:

- the stitching used to sew shut the pockets of your blazers, coats and trousers – now you can use your pockets, should you wish

- the ribbon loops sewn into garments like blouses, skirts and anything sleeveless or off the shoulder. They're useful for retailers to help hang them in store but I can guarantee if you leave them on, they'll sneak out and ruin an otherwise fabulous photo, date, job interview or other significant moment.

- the cotton belt loops you find on the waists of dresses. They indicate where a belt should go and secure the belt in place while hanging in the shop, but their placement is not necessarily where *your* waist is (some of us are long-waisted, some short-waisted, meaning the belt loops may sit at entirely the wrong spot for you). Instead, fix or tie the belt on your natural waist.

Invest in an iron (or a steamer)

I was the designated (paid!) ironer in my household, probably from around the age of fifteen. What I think I liked (and still like) about ironing was the sense of accomplishment and satisfaction I got from taking something messy and unkempt and turning it into something neat and tidy, ready to hang in the wardrobe and be worn.

Keeping your clothing clean and ironed is one of the most fundamental (and easiest) ways to not only increase our clothes' longevity but also make it look and feel expensive. As previously mentioned, I've always been of the opinion that a clean, ironed inexpensive white shirt will look more luxe, stylish and polished than a designer one that is stained and full of wrinkles.

If you find ironing a chore, consider investing in a handheld steamer. There are affordable options available, and they are perfect for when you take something out of the wardrobe that's looking just a little crushed or crinkled and you can't be bothered setting up the ironing board. A steamer has some other great benefits too.

Steaming is gentler on clothing than ironing because it lifts the fibres instead of pressing them down. This reduces the risk of burning or damaging clothes, especially for delicate materials like silk and wool.

Steaming your clothes is environmentally friendly because it can refresh clothing between washes. Less washing helps clothes last longer and also means fewer drycleaner visits. The high heat from a clothes steamer can kill bacteria, allergens and germs that cause odours. This can be especially useful for items that get a bit stinky under the arms or clothing that has been stored for a while.

A handheld steamer is also really useful for getting into all the fiddly places, like a puffed sleeve or a gathered waist, or to smooth out pleating.

Put your clothes away

Tidying up can be the last thing you feel like doing after a long day at work or late night out but just like we know that washing off our make-up before we go to bed is good for our skin, putting away your clothes is good for your personal style. I'm sure we're all guilty at times of using a chair in the bedroom (or perhaps the floor) to throw our clothes between wears with the best intentions to 'put them away later'. But what inevitably happens is that the pile gets bigger and bigger until you no longer know what's in it, and when you do reach for something, it needs an iron or a wash.

When you take a few minutes to hang up or fold and put away your clothing after wearing it, not only will it stay looking fresh for the next time you need it but you're also more likely to recognise if something needs a wash. And just like we discussed earlier, you'll be able to see your wardrobe clearly and choose what to wear with ease.

Launder with care

Take the time to read the care instructions on your garments. It might sound like an obvious piece of advice but it's amazing how many times I've met a client who's ruined a favourite piece of clothing (or someone in their household has) simply by not laundering it properly.

The methods we employ to clean our clothes can also help to extend their life. Putting a polyester blouse on a delicate wash and leaving it to drip dry instead of throwing it in the dryer will ensure the fabric stays wearable for years to come. Dry-cleaning your favourite blazer you bought on the high street will keep it looking brand new. Not washing your new indigo blue jeans with your whites will ensure all your white knickers stay white!

Your style toolkit

If you care enough to invest in a decent wardrobe, you should invest in taking good care of it too. Think of the below as your style saviours – a collection of inexpensive yet essential tools to ensure the contents of your closet stay looking as fresh as the day you first introduced them.

Lint brush

Fluff, dust and especially pet hair can make all clothes, no matter the price, look dishevelled. A lint brush is super handy for removing any build-up and keeping your darker colours looking fresh. There are a few types to choose from, including sticky tape rollers and bristled or silicone reusable brushes.

De-pilling comb

Through everyday wear, knitted garments can pill in the places that receive the most friction, such as under arms, where your crossbody bag rubs, where you sit your toddler on your hip. Even the most expensive woollens pill, so to maintain the look and feel of any knitted piece of clothing, a fabric comb is an essential tool.

Static spray

Static spray is very handy for those moments when your favourite silk dress ends up all 'staticky', sticking to every lump and bump. Static can build up in all sorts of fabrics from silk to nylon and polyester, and when it happens, I've found the best way to combat it is with some good old static spray. My approach is to turn the affected item inside out, lightly spray the static mist in the air and glide the item gently through the mist, almost like you'd walk through a spray of perfume. The static is gone in an instant.

Sewing kit

I think I've owned a sewing kit since early high school, and I highly recommend you keep one on hand. I loved to sew and make my own clothes, so naturally I've always done my own simple alterations, like sewing on a button, darning a sock, taking down a pair of trousers or unpicking the stitching from a jacket pocket. At a minimum, your sewing kit should have a pair of scissors, a seam ripper/unpicker, a needle, dressmaker pins, a measuring tape, a few colours of cotton and perhaps some safety pins.

Dealing with stains

If you're a fan of a good white t-shirt as much as I am – or any high neckline for that matter – then a scarf is going to be your best friend. Let's say you're browsing in a store and your eye lands on a cream silk blouse you absolutely love. It's got a high neckline with a back closure so that the blouse can be taken on and off but you take it from the rack only to find the neckline is covered in someone else's make-up. Unfortunately, this happens a lot. And it's annoying to both you and the retailer, who usually has to get the item laundered or, worse, discard it because they can't sell it.

Use a scarf

Enter the scarf! Many higher-end boutiques have scarves hanging in the changing room for you to place over your face to avoid leaving your make-up on the clothing you're trying on. You've possibly seen these in stores but not known what they were for – don't worry, you're not the only one! It's rare for the retail staff to tell you what they're for. Or, you might have had the experience of using a disposable face scarf in a Japanese department store. I've been told that in Japan, some Uniqlo stores hand you a disposable face covering for you to use when trying on clothes. Genius! While these are designed to be thrown out, there's nothing stopping you from keeping it in your handbag for the next time you go shopping.

To avoid any make-up transfer on your own clothing, I recommend keeping a covering at home that you use to put on and take off any item of clothing that goes over your head, especially one that has a fitted neckline or is a light colour.

Simply place the covering over your head and face (you want to ensure your entire face is covered), put your garment over your head as normal, then remove the scarf to reveal a stain-free collar or neckline. Do the same thing to take the garment off.

Not only will the scarf prevent you from staining your clothing, but it also means you might not have to wash the item after every wear. It's always annoyed me when I have to wash something like a white t-shirt just because the neckline is stained but the rest of the garment is fine. Less washing is not only good for the environment but also good for the longevity of your clothes.

My scarf of choice is an inexpensive polyester one that can be thrown in the wash every now and then. The 'slipperiness' of the fabric means the clothes glide over my head easily. The size of the scarf is important too – too small and it might not cover your entire face but too big and you'll get frustrated with all the excess fabric.

Using a scarf is also a great tip when you're trying on any online purchases that you may end up returning. I bet you'd appreciate it if whoever tried on the item before you did the same. I always take a scarf shopping with me and I now pack one when going on holiday.

Use hairspray

Another simple hack for avoiding stains on the collars of your light-coloured clothing is hairspray. You may have successfully avoided transferring your make-up while getting dressed but what about during the rest of the day as your skin goes through its natural process of cell shedding? Hairspray around your neckline will act as a 'barrier' between your skin and your clothing. The trick is to let the hairspray dry before you put your clothes on, and to use a light hairspray rather than a sticky lacquer. As well as necklines, cuffs can be a trouble spot for other stains, so try the hairspray trick here too.

Common stains to avoid

Other common products that may cause stains on your clothing include fake tan, sunscreen, deodorant and body lotion. We may not always be able to avoid the transfer of these products but we can take precautions to reduce the chances of it happening.

Sunscreen and deodorant, for example, both have an annoying habit of leaving unsightly yellow stains on our clothing, often impossible to get rid of once we discover them. A simple thing you can do to minimise this happening is to ensure you let your sunscreen and deodorant completely dry and fully absorb into your skin before you get dressed.

The quicker you get on to any stains, the better. Try using a baby wipe to gently remove any marks. Retailers will often try this on clothing that's been marked in store, and it's definitely worth trying yourself. If that doesn't work, try to launder the affected item as quickly as you can by first applying a pre-stain remover and then washing it in cold water with like colours. If you've not tried the Sard Wonder pre-treater stain stick, I suggest you do!

How to remove unwanted smells

You're heading into a job interview, and naturally you're nervous. Your tummy is full of butterflies, and you can feel yourself sweating under your arms as you wait for your turn to be called into the office. As soon as you sit down, you relax. The panellists make you feel comfortable and at ease, the butterflies settle and the perspiration stops. When you get home and change out of your interview outfit, you give the underarms of your blouse a sniff. It's a bit 'whiffy' but you only wore it for a couple of hours and really don't want to wash it or, worse, have to take it to the drycleaner.

Here are three of my top smell-removal tips. Regardless of what method you use, the results will mean less laundering of your clothes and it will also save you money on your dry-cleaning bills.

Use Febreze

I shared a hack for this on my Instagram that was well received by most, and controversial for some. For many years, I've used Febreze fabric spray to remove underarm odour from my clothes between washes. It works! Febreze is a deodoriser, designed to remove odours caused by pet mishaps, food spillages and anything else leaving unpleasant odours, including clothes. I always do a spot test on more delicate fabrics like silk, mostly to check if the Febreze leaves a mark once dry. It never has. I turn my garments inside out and spray the Febreze onto the affected area, then leave to dry overnight. The next morning, it smells as fresh as a daisy!

Use vodka

Now, for those of you averse to using chemicals, I have a more 'natural' approach to removing underarm odour: vodka! Pure, old-fashioned (unflavoured) vodka. Apparently, this hack has been used in the theatre world for years when stage costumes cannot be cleaned from one performance to the next. If you can spare a little from the liquor cabinet, pour a small amount into a spray bottle. As with the Febreze, flip your garment inside out, give the affected area a good spray, leave to dry and voila! Smelly underarms be gone.

Use a steamer

A third method is to employ a handheld steamer to the area to help freshen up the garment. This is a super convenient way to deodorise the underarms of your favourite tee between wears and my preferred method for my silk dresses and blazers.

How to protect your shoes

Get Topy'd

Whether you've got a very healthy 'shoerobe' or a few pairs on high rotation, you need to know what a Topy is: a rubber sole glued to the bottom of shoes to protect them from wear and tear. Essentially, it's a sole attached to the sole.

Some leather-soled shoes will come with an in-built rubber sole but many do not. That's where your local cobbler comes in. I have had many leather-soled shoes Topy'd, and some non-leather ones too. Here's why: a leather-soled shoe will start to wear down at both the tips and the heel. As this happens, we risk damage to the upper leather, which can tear and discolour. If you've ever worn pointed-toe shoes, you'll be able to relate. As the sole wears down, those once beautiful points start to look a bit worse for wear. Adding a rubber Topy will help protect the tips of your shoes from wearing down and damaging the upper leather. And a cobbler can attach a rubber heel to protect the heels from wearing down.

Over the years I've also had a few pairs of boots with a synthetic sole. They didn't 'wear down' so much as simply split in two! I was able to rescue them with a Topy sole, which not only gave me another few seasons' wear but also made them much more weatherproof. The added bonus is that a Topy also provides a non-slippery surface, which, depending on your terrain, can be good during rain, frost and grime.

The ultimate benefit that a Topy provides is longevity. A Topy can be replaced time and time again, prolonging the life of your shoes and continuing to protect the upper leather (or other fabric) from wear and tear.

Waterproof your shoes

Protecting your shoes with waterproof protector can extend the life of shoes made from delicate materials like suede. It can also improve the performance of technical shoes like hiking boots. While good-quality pairs will come with some protection, once they've been out in the elements a few times, and/or if you run them through the wash, it never hurts to add an extra layer of protective spray. Likewise, regularly polishing your leather shoes will keep them looking good and improve their durability.

How to protect your feet

There are so many tools at our disposal to make wearing shoes more comfortable, and I know how important comfort is to most of us. Here are my favourite tools for everything feet related.

Toe covers

If you're like me and suffer from blistering on your toes in enclosed shoes that you wear without socks, you need to know about toe covers. They are brilliant! They protect your tootsies and, let's be honest, they also help stop your shoes from smelling (to a degree). I wear these covers with shoes that don't require socks or pantihose – think ballet flats, loafers, pumps, et cetera. They're completely invisible when worn with a lower vamp shoe.

Gel cushions

There's a reason most shoe stores have an accessories section right near the counter, and it's not just to upsell you into buying more products! Gel cushions, designed to wear under the soles of your feet, are something I recommend to all my clients. First, they provide support for the balls of your feet, particularly when wearing heels. Second, they're great for helping stop your foot from slipping forward in strappy sandals. And third, they're a strategic way to make a slightly too-big shoe fit better. By taking up a bit more space in the toe box, they push your foot back into the heel of the shoe, avoiding it slipping off as you walk.

You can also use these self-adhesive cushions on any part of your shoes that rub because they're easy to chop into any shape and size. I've used them as heel grips to stop my heels from blistering, on the back of buckles to stop them rubbing and on the back of ankle straps to keep them in place.

Knowing these hacks won't necessarily improve your personal style but they will help you put your best foot forward (with your Topy and toe covers) when it comes to getting dressed, helping you go about your day feeling confident and comfortable!

A few more favourite hacks

I couldn't finish this chapter without sharing a few more of my most-trusted hacks related to making your clothes work for you. These ones are less about wear and tear and more about looking your fabulous best in other ways but they're no less valuable.

Check the hem allowance

If you're vertically 'enhanced' like me and find that pants are often not quite long enough, then a false hem might come to the rescue. Again, it's such a simple thing to do but many people don't know what one is.

Pretty much every item of clothing has a hem but depending on the garment, that hem may be quite small or quite generous. A tailor can take down the hem to achieve the maximum length by adding a false hem to the garment. This involves attaching a separate strip of material (your tailor will have this) to add length to a garment. This is not visible, since it is part of the material that is turned up under the hem. But the difference to how a garment looks on the body is obvious.

How to maintain your hemline

If you're someone who sometimes needs to get trousers and jeans shortened, did you know that you can ask for the original hem to be retained? This is not always necessary, such as with a simple pair of trousers, but most blue jeans have some contrasting features on the hem, such as colour variation, fading or distressing, which you'll likely want to keep. The hem is part of the jean's DNA, giving it some personality. When a tailor simply chops the jeans and sews a new hem, it can ruin the original feel of the jeans, sometimes making an expensive pair look cheap. Asking for the original hem to be reattached will cost a little extra but will ensure authenticity and disguise the fact that you've had them tailored.

How to keep your sleeves up

Another wardrobe game changer for me has been a simple tool to help my jacket sleeves (or any sleeve, really) stay up. Sleeve guards, sleeve bands, sleeve garters – whatever the name – allow you to roll up the sleeves of a jacket and position them exactly where you want to, without fiddling or adjusting them throughout the day. Unlike a hair elastic, they're gentler and kinder on your clothes and they won't cut off your circulation!

As a styling tool, these also allow you to manipulate your outfit to create interesting layers. You might use them to hold up your jacket sleeves to expose the great cuffs on your shirt, or to expose your forearms to help balance out an oversized outfit.

And I have another use for them. Try them on the hem of your pants! I love to use my sleeve bands to turn a straight leg trouser into more of a jogger style. They work particularly well on light fabrics and can completely transform a pant into a completely new style, for a completely different purpose!

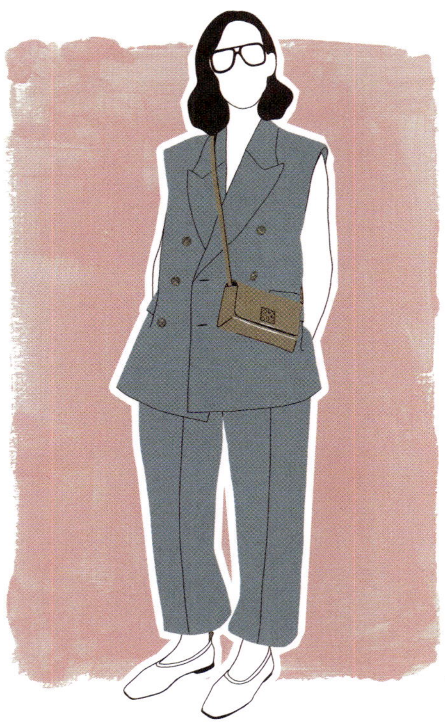

Fasten your coat belts

Have you ever got home only to discover you've lost the belt on your favourite coat? Belted coats can look really chic, highlighting the waist but most of the time when we throw on our trench or winter coat for the commute to work, to pop out to get our morning coffee or throw it over our activewear for the school run, we don't use the belt.

Enter the coat belt-fasten hack! This trick means you'll never lose a belt again and you can still use the belt when required *and* avoid the messy, bulky 'back tie' we so often default to. Loop the belt through the belt loops, then fasten it to itself (rather than tying it). You're still able to use the belt when needed but there is no chance that belt is going anywhere. The bonus is that you create a nice, smooth line across the back of the coat, making it look more elevated and more comfortable to sit in.

Look after your wardrobe

Clearly personal style is important to you or you wouldn't be reading this book! Given how much effort you put into your clothing collection, I hope you can see that treating your key pieces with the care they deserve will allow them a special place in your wardrobe for years to come. And this even goes for your seasonal crush pieces too. With these hacks at your fingertips, you'll be able to look and feel your best as you head out for your day, comfortable and secure from head to toe.

If you care enough to *invest* in a decent wardrobe, you should invest in taking *good care of it*, too.

15. SHOWCASE BOUNDLESS STYLE

One of the most wonderful things about using social media, which we leant into in Chapter 2, is the diversity it has brought us. Back in the day, our ideas were limited to what we were fed through localised, mainstream media, whereas these days we can collect, curate and follow people and style from across the globe. This has taught us the beauty of embracing looks and styles that suit every body at every age.

As a passionate advocate for self-expression and ageless style, I love celebrating how our personal style can evolve and strengthen as we progress through life. As a woman goes through life, her outlook, interests, body shape and lifestyle change. Naturally, her personal style changes along with it. This is why I encourage all my clients, from a young age, to be less concerned with being 'on trend' or 'fitting in' and instead care more about embracing their unique identity and cultivating a style that represents the person we are and want others to see. Personal style is ageless, and I believe that someone's age should never determine what they wear, where they shop or what their style personality should be.

What is timeless style?

If you've ever searched the term 'timeless style', you'll no doubt have been served images of women with a very particular look – likely wearing some variation of a white cotton shirt, tailored trousers, loafers, a neat-fitting trench or blazer and a handbag. This particular style is often 'encouraged' as the 'age-appropriate' style for women of a certain age. Yet, while I (and many of my friends and clients) fit that vintage, I typically don't see a lot of this! Instead, I see women of all ages owning their style, shopping wherever they please and wearing whatever they want.

I'm glad this is becoming the norm because it wasn't always that way.

In my early forties, I started a series of panel discussions to open up the conversation around fashion and ageism. I had observed that the older my clients got, the stronger their interest in fashion became. Age hadn't diminished their passion – it had enhanced it. Many had more time and income at their disposal compared with their younger selves, and they wanted to put them to good use. They certainly didn't want to be overlooked by the fashion industry, feel dismissed by their favourite brands or submit to a version of what a woman is supposed to wear at a 'certain age'.

My style philosophy is about embracing who you are at every age, whether you're just beginning to consider your style or are rejoicing in its fifth evolution. This chapter, like the rest of this book, is not about what you should wear for your age. It is about how and why you should continue to wear clothes that express your style personality and continue to feel your best. If that so happens to be a look that many might describe as 'classic', so be it – but even that doesn't mean you have to look boring or conservative!

Fashion inspiration before social media

Before the rise of social media platforms, there were blogs, where everyday people shared aspects of their lives, including their passion for style, regardless of their location, age, size or budget. Fashion blogs became a creative outlet for people who lived and breathed fashion to showcase their style to a broad audience. Suddenly, fashion didn't feel like a secret club, only privy to those on the inside.

Before blogs, we'd had to wait for our favourite monthly fashion magazines to get our inspiration. The magazines of the 1980s and 1990s featured almost exclusively models, usually in their early twenties, showcasing upcoming collections and new trends. And because they were models, they usually had a singular body type and often just one skin tone.

To think back and realise that most of us were not represented in any way is quite appalling. We've come a long way but no doubt there's a long way to go. While the fashion world of magazines and catwalks may still be littered with tall, thin models (older models are now more common but they're still mostly thin), it is no longer our *only* source of style inspiration, and that is a very good thing.

Fashion magazines, campaigns and catwalks will always have their place in the fashion industry for showcasing new trends and supporting the designers who create them, but how lucky are we that today we have more options for consuming fashion and style via social media. Now, we can see our favourite brands on women who represent a more accurate cross-section of the 'everyday woman'.

Become ageless

In today's world of social media, we have broadened our definitions of what and who is 'in fashion'. Nonetheless, one category that remains under-represented in this space is older women. From the models on the catwalk to those featured in advertising campaigns and online imagery, to the content creators engaged by brands, there is a lot that can be done to improve visibility.

Our love for fashion, for style and for feeling great in our clothes doesn't age just because we do. If anything, it gets stronger as we come to know ourselves better and feel more confident in our choices. Instead of ignoring our instincts, we lean into them.

Style helps us transcend society's arbitrary limits, such as the social norms that have traditionally told us no. Think of how many times you've read or heard that 'women can't do x, y, z', 'they're too old', 'she's too short, too big, too this, too that'. The right outfit has the ability to transcend these constructs – it can uplift, inspire, empower, *transform*.

Clothing is a powerful tool that can give us the confidence to face the day and express our personality, and age should never determine that, nor limit it. We can't stop the ageing process, but we can keep our style ageless. I truly believe that knowing your style, owning your style and feeling your style is the biggest antidote for ageing.

Style helps us *transcend* society's arbitrary limits.

How to evolve your style

Your style personality words will shift and change throughout life; that's natural and to be expected. A desire to dress 'grungy' in your twenties won't necessarily align with how you want your clothing to feel in your fifties. But equally, don't assume that you *must* let go of your style words just because you're older. Your interpretation of the same word can change instead.

As an example, I want to explore a style descriptor typically associated with 'ageless style'. Using real-life examples of women I've worked with, I want to show you how it can apply at any age. In fashion terms, 'timeless' refers to clothing that is not affected by the passage of time or changes in trends. While some people will have a strong liking for 'timeless' styles, colours and silhouettes, what about the rest of us? Are we all supposed to conform to 'looking the same' as we age in order to be considered stylish?

When you search the term 'timeless style' on Pinterest, it becomes abundantly clear how the algorithm defines it. On the day I searched it, it meant:

- a beige blazer
- white cotton shirt
- black straight-leg pants
- a camel knee-length trench
- black loafers
- tan ballet flats.

All these items are indeed timeless, and a wardrobe full of these pieces may appeal to you wholeheartedly. But I would argue they can appeal to you at twenty-five, forty-five or seventy-five! Whether or not you want to wear items like this is determined by your style personality, not your age. Let's look closer at some of these timeless items.

The timeless trench

Both Caterina and Freya have classic styles but each interpret the word 'timeless' in different ways. Caterina leans more heavily into a classic 'timeless' style, whereas Freya prefers a more creative approach. Different ages, different style personalities, different versions of 'timeless'.

Caterina

Caterina is in her thirties. She loves to keep things simple when it comes to her outfits, including her choice of colours. Her wardrobe consists mostly of navy, camel, white and grey. She admires the style of Hollywood actors past and present like Audrey Hepburn, Jennifer Aniston and Reese Witherspoon. Her go-to wardrobe staple is her camel trench coat. Classic in style, length, fit and fabric, it can be thrown over everything from her slim-leg jeans and loafers on the weekend to her pencil skirts and blouses for work. She likes the timelessness of her trench coat as it aligns with her classic, understated style and her preference for getting value and wearability from her wardrobe. Caterina adds flair to her otherwise timeless wardrobe by adding pops of colour through scarfs, shoes and handbags. She hunts for these in vintage stores, which gives her outfits individuality while channelling her idols.

Freya

Freya is in her sixties. Though a creative type working in the arts, she is a minimalist in terms of her colour palette and wears only navy, camel, white and grey. She loves the simplicity of having what she refers to as a 'uniform' for her everyday life, and this timeless colour palette allows her to mix and match her wardrobe with ease. She also owns a camel trench coat. Her trench is relaxed on the body, falls to mid-calf, and is made of a patent faux leather with a snakeskin finish. Freya loves the uniqueness of her trench, and the creative vibe it adds to her classic yet contemporary wardrobe of navy pants, camel loafers and handbags.

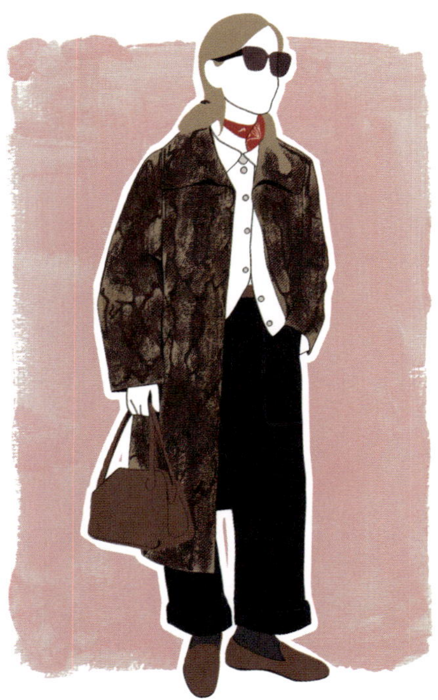

The timeless black loafer

Janice, Yan and Mila all love their black loafers – a shoe style that stands the test of time. Loafers are timeless wardrobe staples, and yet, as each of these examples shows, the wide range of variations available make it possible to find a black loafer that perfectly expresses your unique style and lifestyle.

Janice

Style personality: *timeless*, *modern*, *edgy*.

Janice, 71, is a retired author who has recently moved to a rural town inhabited by many artists and known for its thriving creative industries. She had always loved fashion and during her career had worn a lot of independent designers, especially those who focused on draping, asymmetric hemlines, bold silhouettes and lots of black. Janice had a strong sense of personal style and, while her lifestyle had changed, she still wanted to look and feel like herself in her new home environment.

Since retiring and moving from the city, Janice had little need (or patience) for her amazing collection of statement high heels. She didn't want to wear sneakers – they just didn't feel like her – but she'd succumbed to them because she wasn't sure what other options were available.

I suggested we look at a black loafer, a 'timeless' item but in a style that would align with her other style personality words of 'modern' and 'edgy'. Because Janice had been used to wearing heels, I showed her a loafer with a platform sole. She instantly loved the idea. The shoes also had a large, brushed silver buckle, white contrast stitching and were made of a patent mock-croc leather.

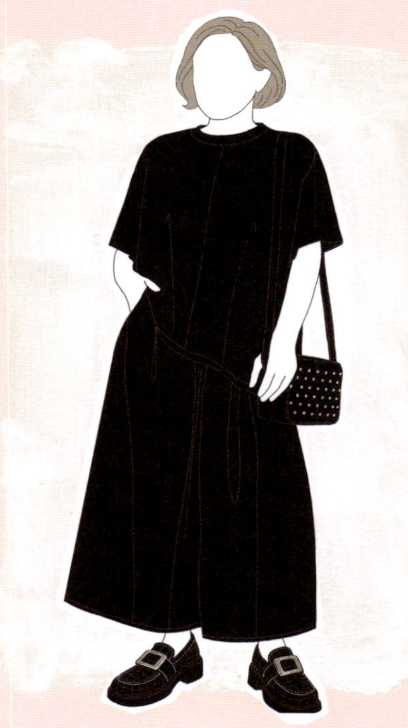

Yan

Style personality: *timeless*, *sporty*, *androgynous*.

Yan, 29, runs an advertising company that is high paced, competitive and dynamic. Her office is located in an old warehouse in the inner city. Yan sets the tone and encourages her staff to dress as they please – no suits required, though her own suits are rather iconic among her colleagues and clients. She wears oversized, bold, vintage suits in bright colours that she dresses down with sneakers, rugby jerseys or sports t-shirts and baseball caps.

When I met Yan, she too was needing help to fill a gap in her shoe wardrobe. She had plenty of sneakers but she needed a more polished option for an upcoming international stakeholder meeting where she knew they just wouldn't cut it.

I introduced her to a black loafer with a white rubber sole. These felt just right. The white sole was in keeping with her signature sporty sneaker style, while the strong, square toe was a nod to her androgynous aesthetic.

Mila

Style personality: *timeless*, *casual*, *conservative*.

Mila, 46, works part-time as a carer for children with disabilities and is a mother of three. While she always likes to make an effort and look put together, she's not really into fashion, so prefers to buy timeless pieces that she can wear for many years. She is happy for her work and everyday wardrobe to be one and the same, as long as her clothes are comfortable, functional and practical. For Mila, it made sense to develop a 'uniform' of sorts: striped merino jumpers, black slim pants, black shoes, black bag and a black quilted vest when required.

When I met Mila, her black shoes were chunky, black 'walking' sneakers. While they were comfortable and appropriate for work, she was feeling a bit unsure about them when spending time around other women whose style she admired as being a little more 'modern'.

I suggested we try a classic black loafer. We tried on a few different styles

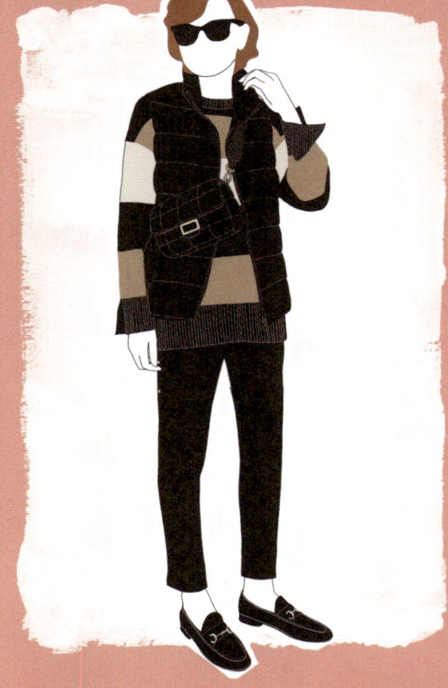

including some with leather soles and rubber soles; some made of patent leather and cracked leather; and some with features like tassels, horse bits and fringing. Mila's preference was a classic, timeless black loafer with a comfortable rubber sole, no bells and whistles. They worked perfectly with her classic uniform but she felt more put together and stylish in them over her sneakers.

An edgy classic

As the loafers example showed, it is quite possible to twist a so-called 'classic' item to suit your style personality. The word 'classic' is used prolifically in fashion, especially to describe a personal style aesthetic that is clean, neutral and tailored. As the definition implies, a classic style is often used to describe pieces that are less likely to date and so stand the test of time. But as Sian shows, one person's interpretation of 'classic' will be different from the next.

Sian

Style personality: *sexy*, *edgy*, *simple*, *classic*.

We've met urban-dwelling Sian before. Sian's style is edgy, sexy and monochromatic. She wears clothing that is fitted rather than oversized, preferring to show shape at the waist, even in casual outfits. Sian's style is simple, preferring clean lines and classic silhouettes.

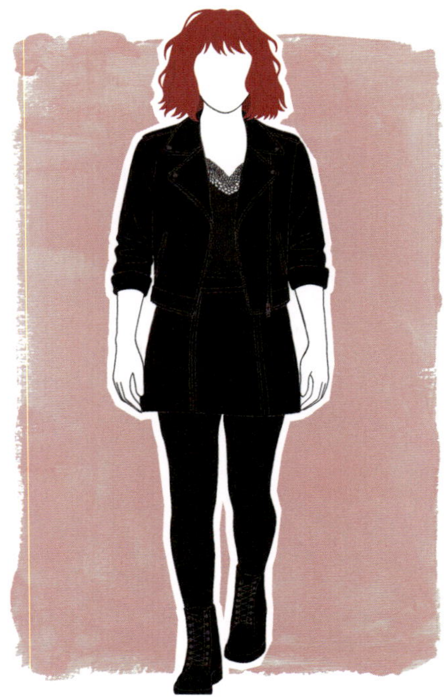

Sian's wardrobe consists almost entirely of black clothes and accessories, and because this is her style preference, my job is not to try to convince her to add colour but to work with what she owns and feels her best in. Although far from conservative, the word 'classic' could still be used to describe her black combat boots, high-heeled ankle boots, black cardigan, black leather jacket, black skinny jeans and her favourite black leather pencil skirt.

Why? Because her wardrobe is full of timeless pieces but with an edge. Her clothes are simple, not driven by trends and are classic in shape. Her black winter coat, which she's owned for years, features unique gunmetal buttons that nip her in at the waist. It neatly frames her shoulders and it falls to just above the knee. She likes to add a statement black belt with gunmetal eyelets all over to emphasise her waist even more. Simple, edgy and classic in style, sexy in fit.

When styling her wardrobe for summer, Sian enjoys throwing on a simple black silk slip dress with black open-toe mules and a black bucket bag. In autumn she transitions this look by adding her black leather biker jacket and switching out her mules for ankle boots and tights. Sian's is an unconventional classic style but classic, nonetheless.

We can't stop the ageing process, but we can keep our style *ageless*.

A new approach to timeless inspiration

As we discussed in Chapter 2, social media can be a useful source of inspiration and has really helped bring fashion to the people. Fashion these days is far more broadly represented with style mavens from all ages and walks of life readily feeding us their take on how best to dress. I love the inspiration social media offers but, like anything, if consumed unchecked it can have its downsides.

As such, I think it's important to have a discussion around how to use it best, to serve our needs in the most positive, productive way. I do appreciate that social media is not perfect and it's not always a safe space. People can be cruel. Over time, I've curated my feed to become a welcoming haven that encourages and motivates me. It's a source of positivity, inspiration and enjoyment, and I want the same for you! Inspiration can come from many sources and the only person who can truly judge whether that content is of value is you. To help you curate a social media feed that inspires, uplifts and motivates you, I've come up with some guidelines.

Follow accounts that:

- make you feel good about yourself

- inspire your personal style (regardless of the creator's age, gender, size, location and budget)

- inspire you to look at your wardrobe in new ways

- promote creativity and trying new things

- offer value you trust.

Unfollow accounts that:

- leave you questioning your self-worth

- are driven by 'rules'

- are just trying to sell you stuff.

Below are some examples of accounts I follow on social media that adhere to the above guidelines. If you're not on social media, you can apply the same advice to blogs you read, podcasts you listen to, newsletters you subscribe to, magazines you buy or the TV programs you watch.

My inspirations

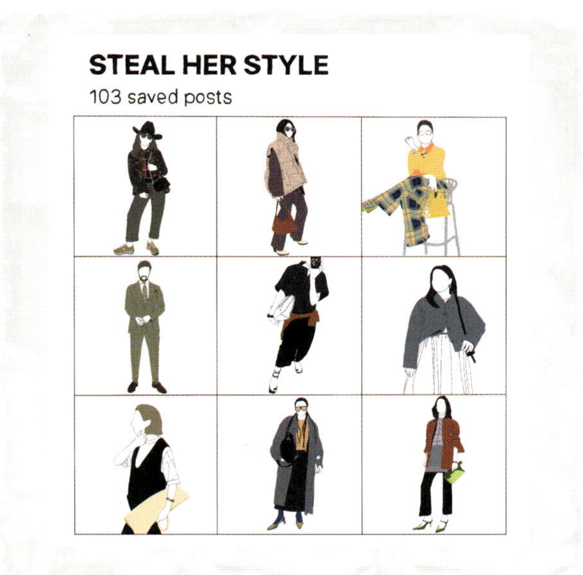

Ageless-style advocate, eclectic style, storyteller

There's something about this woman I follow that mesmerises me – she 'stops the scroll' every time. Yes, she's a great storyteller but she's also got a great attitude towards ageing and wearing whatever she wants. Her personal style doesn't particularly resonate with me; neither does her lifestyle. But her ability to 'get dressed' while telling a story and leaving the viewer with not only a pretty cool outfit combination but a subliminal message is quite the talent!

She inspires me to be my true self, to take risks with my style and to please myself and nobody else. It makes me so happy to see a beautiful woman in her sixties embracing the body she's got and ageing naturally. I admire her confidence to put herself out there, and to be seen.

Entrepreneur, mother of three, designer 'clothes horse'

This woman has great style and an insane wardrobe that I love, but while we're both style entrepreneurs, our lifestyles are completely different. She has three children, lives in a different country, flies first class and spends a lot of time in the Hamptons. And her clothing is expensive – like, very expensive – entire outfits of international designer labels (think The Row, Bottega, Prada, Jil Sander, Loewe, et cetera). But there's an ease and subtleness to her not-so-obvious luxury looks.

I am inspired by her style choices in creating outfits that are simple, polished and timeless. And while I cannot afford to wear head-to-toe designer outfits, she has influenced how I feel about obvious designer branding and therefore my purchasing habits. Her style also prompts me to reflect on my own wardrobe and to try new combinations that create more 'ease' and simplicity when I feel like it. Her style, while unattainable for my budget, still provides me with inspiration when considering new pieces for my wardrobe from brands that fall more comfortably in my price bracket.

British digital creator – eclectic, vintage aesthetic

I'm not a big second-hand shopper (sorry, Mum) but I do often re-think my old pieces by exploring small tweaks that might make something feel new again. This creator inspires me with her use of colour. She thinks outside the square with her outfit combinations and challenges the traditional approach to personal style 'after a certain age'. She wears a lot of second-hand items and loves to upcycle old clothes by altering them for a brand-new look.

While our personal styles, age and body shapes are quite different, what I gain from following her is a greater sense of playfulness and experimentation. Her energy is always uplifting: she often dances while getting dressed, and she's always smiling in her reels and posts. She takes me on a journey that is both unpredictable and engaging, and I always watch until the end for the ensuing outcome.

Charismatic male content creator from the USA

You might be surprised that I follow quite a few men for style inspiration. This one in particular has a seamless way of speaking to camera and educating his audience. I follow him because he inspires me to create content in a simple, formulated way, with great visual representations to back that up.

I also like his approach to building outfits. He accessorises in unexpected ways, taking what initially looks to be a pretty classic outfit to a more interesting place, and his explanations make me think about my own wardrobe. What inspires me most about him is his ability to make style simple and accessible to everyone. He's not selling me stuff, he's teaching me, nurturing me, always supportive and never judgemental.

Petite fashion designer from Sweden

What can I say? I'm obsessed. This woman wears her own designs 99 per cent of the time, which I love, but cannot afford to wear head to toe. Nor do I want to – I like to wear lots of different brands. But the aesthetic she creates with her outfits – their look, feel and ease – speaks to me. Following her has made me look at my own style very differently. She's a straight shooter:

no BS. She hates rules. Following her reminds and reassures me of my own thoughts on style.

She's created a following of like-minded people who align with those values and feelings about personal style, and it's a great, supportive community. So, while my own personal style doesn't always align with hers, my values do.

Curvy mid-size influencer from the UK, minimalist

Sometimes I follow people not because I'm drawn to their personal style but I like their approach to styling. This woman is a completely different body shape to me, is much younger and showcases a lot of 'high street' fashion on her account. But what I love about her is that she challenges typical beliefs of how a plus-size woman should dress. She wears a mix of fitted and baggy clothes, experiments with tailored and oversized silhouettes on her body, and only wears flat shoes. And she always looks great. She confidently shares pictures of herself in swimwear on holidays, which encourages me to feel less self-conscious and more comfortable in my own skin.

Seeing a fuller-figured woman with great style sharing her outfits provides me with great perspective and inspiration when it comes to styling my clients too. I'm also able to share these accounts with them so they can see their own body type represented in a positive way.

I don't have to *love or like* everything they say, do or wear, and that's okay.

What to be wary of

While the examples of people I've mentioned are varied, the outcome is the same: they each inspire me in a positive way. I don't have to love or like everything they say, do or wear, and that's okay. What they don't do is prescribe to me how I should dress, telling me the '10 must-have items to add to your wardrobe this season!' or bombarding me with messages about how to look slimmer, curvier, younger or whatever attribute might be 'trending' right now.

Influencers are called influencers for a reason. That term has never particularly sat well with me but I understand its relevance and application. The whole point of my social media is to influence my followers; whether to have more self-confidence, to try new colour combinations, to use my styling services or to buy the pieces I promote when collaborating with brands. But I have always created my content wearing my stylist hat – and, come to think of it, my teaching hat too.

The accounts you follow on social media should be ones that inspire you, challenge you and help you with your personal style in a positive way. They should encourage your creativity, foster your individuality and champion your sense of style no matter your size, shape, age or budget.

If an account you follow entices you to constantly overconsume, leaving you guilt ridden and with a wardrobe full of clothes you don't wear, then I would argue it's time to unfollow. If a creator you follow, through no fault of their own, leaves you feeling less worthy, not trendy enough, not wealthy enough, not good enough, I would also unfollow.

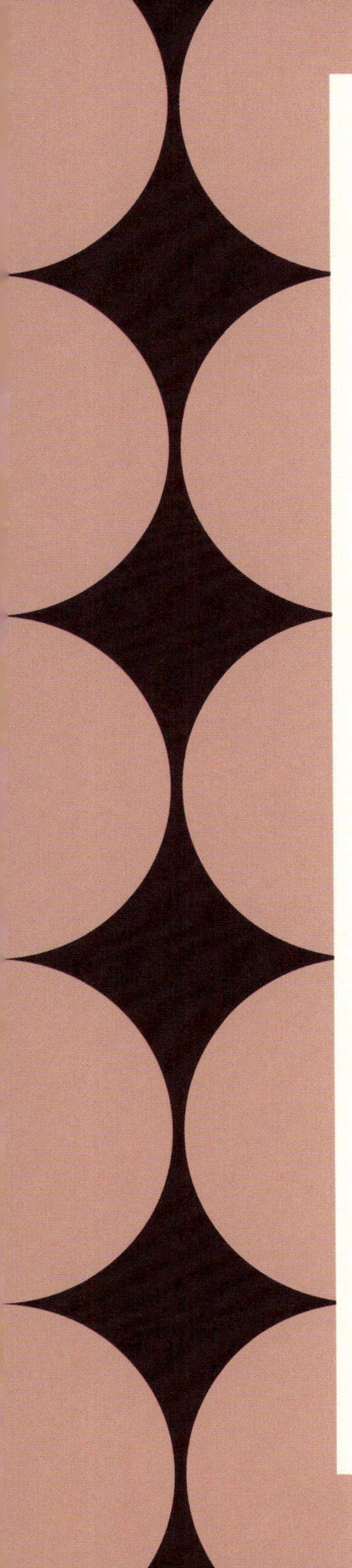

Activity: Curate your feed

What you need:
pen and paper
your preferred social media platform

Grab a notebook and pen, and write down the top three to five accounts you follow, whose posts you regularly like, comment on or save, leaving some space under each one. Once you've come up with your list, take a few minutes to scroll each of their feeds and view their content. Just theirs.

Make some notes about how each account's content makes you *feel*. Not what you learn from each of them but what it is about them that makes you feel more confident with your own personal style, age, body shape, size, hair colour or your shopping habits.

You can use this task to do two things:

1. reinforce how you want social media to benefit you

2. help you unfollow or avoid following accounts that do not align with your values.

Just like we pick and choose the people in our lives who we want to spend our valuable time with, you can pick and choose who you want to follow. You wouldn't hang around someone who constantly made you feel insecure about your body or self-conscious about your choice of clothing, or who pressured you to buy something every time you caught up.

We should have people in our lives who accept us for who we are, who champion our individuality and encourage us to be the best versions of ourselves – and I think about social media the same way. Think of social media as the friendship group you curate to hang out and have fun with, not the mean girls from high school.

Style beyond limits

I've purposely placed this chapter towards the end of the book for an important reason. To me, boundless style means style without limits: age, body shape, lifestyle or other. Style is something that should enhance your life, not detract from it. If you reach a point where you're finding your style choices restrictive, take it as a sign to review. Part of what keeps us looking fresh and feeling timeless is our willingness to continue to embrace change and adapt our style to suit our life throughout its different stages.

Age is irrelevant to the advice and principles I share. Your age does not determine your style personality, your wardrobe purpose or your Three Cs. Our age is insignificant when it comes to organising our wardrobes, shopping like a pro or building outfits. Your age is inconsequential when embracing your shape, discovering your colours or using social media to seek inspiration and new looks to experiment with.

By sharing these examples of women I've worked with and my varied social media style inspirations, I hope to challenge the stereotype of how we are supposed to dress 'for our age'. I yearn that one day soon I will search #agelessstyle and see a wider variety of style mavens, just like the ones we've met here, wearing all sorts of fabulous clothes.

Timeless style is not a rulebook for us to follow when we reach a certain age, and it's not about adhering to a dress code where classic neutrals and sensible shoes are in, and bold colours and impractical shoes are out! Regardless of our age, fashion should be fun, interesting and ever changing. Your self-confidence and joy in expressing yourself should be the decisive factor behind whether you've chosen to wear a miniskirt or a sequin jacket, nothing else! We should continue to try new things, take risks and evolve our personal style. As Iris Apfel once famously said, 'When the fun goes out of dressing, you might as well be dead.' Good style is emphatically ageless, and when it comes to personal style, the best is yet to come.

16. TRAVEL IN STYLE

I love to travel, and I'm sure you do too – so many amazing sights and magical experiences! But have you ever looked back at holiday photos and thought to yourself, 'I hate what I'm wearing'? It can really take the shine off an otherwise wonderful holiday and the memories you created.

Then there's the packing, which I used to hate. Whether it was for a midwinter long weekend away with friends or a European summer holiday, the task of deciding what to take used to stress me out. What was the weather going to be? How much walking was I going to do? Where would we be going out for dinner? What would everyone else be wearing? For years, I got it wrong – very wrong. I'd pack the wrong shoes or too many shoes, not enough layers or too many layers, and I'd always overpack. I would go on these holidays and feel very much 'out of place', and often hot and bothered – literally!

The good news is that I've now worked out some trusty methods to make packing easier and to help you feel great while travelling – and I'm going to share them with you.

Dress to feel like you

I have come to the realisation that no matter the location, the climate or the company, I want to dress in a way that feels like me. My goal is to wear clothes that meet the criteria – suitable for the weather, planned activities and cultural sensitivities – but still reflect my style personality. This is the first secret to successful travel dressing. For years, I felt like a bit of an imposter, dressing to fit in rather than dressing to be myself, feeling self-conscious in a new city or country because I wasn't expressing my true self through my clothes. I would not only pack clothing that didn't align with my style but also outfits that I simply wouldn't wear at home. For example, on a hot day walking around Melbourne, I would never choose a strappy dress that exposed a lot of skin – that would make me feel anxious about getting sunburnt and, worse, skin cancer. Equally, I wouldn't wear a pair of cut-off denim shorts on a hot day to go to work, out for brunch or to a museum, but for some reason I'd pack them to do literally the same things in another place. Inevitably, I never felt like myself on holiday.

Travelling is great but it can also be really challenging. New countries, different languages, unfamiliar customs – it can be a lot! Dressing and feeling like yourself can be the one thing you have control of in a new environment and can help you go about your day with greater confidence and enjoyment. And I guarantee you'll look back at your photos and love what you were wearing.

Of course, it's important to factor in things like being comfortable for long days of sightseeing and having options to keep you warm, cool or protected from the sun. And for the purpose of this chapter, we're not talking about adventure holidays like an African safari or an overland hiking adventure! These types of holidays require disciplined packing where practicality and functionality carry more importance than style.

When packing to go on a holiday, aim to create a curated capsule of the things you love to wear and align the contents of your suitcase with your style personality. Whether you're packing for an overseas city adventure, a weekend getaway to the coast or a relaxing week in a countryside villa, if you use your style words to guide you, you really can't go wrong.

Whether you're going out for dinner, to an art gallery, window shopping or attending a festival, the clothing that you pack and the outfits that you wear should be what you'd wear to do the same things at home (with the exception of cultural sensitivities such as covering your shoulders in certain locations where you might wear a tank or strappy top at home). If you wouldn't wear leggings out for lunch, hiking shoes to go shopping or a puffer jacket to the theatre, then why wear them to do so on holiday?

I now pack a dress that covers my back and decolletage, is a midi length and is made of a lightweight cotton that is cool and breathable and perfect for days when there will be incidental sun exposure. Instead of denim shorts, I pack full-length silk or linen pants that feel chic, polished and airy. Just as I dress to feel like myself at home on a hot summer's day, I dress to feel like myself on a summer holiday.

Repeating outfits

Often, we overpack because we want to ensure we have different outfits for different occasions and purposes. But guess what? When you're on holidays, you're not in your usual environment, seeing the same work colleagues every day, hanging out with the same friends every weekend or bumping into the same school mums every day at pick-up. You can repeat outfits more than you might at home, saving space in your suitcase – it'll be lighter too!

Pack outfits that you feel great in and wear them more than once – not everything needs to be washed after one wear, and you might have access to laundry facilities depending on the length of your trip. And even if you are taking photographs of yourself every day and posting them on social media, who cares if you are wearing the same outfit on more than one occasion?

While by now you know I am not a rule follower, I do use various guidelines for travel packing, simply because they help me limit my choices. Though I can't pretend to have invented these myself, I have tried and tested them all and here are a few of my favourites. They've alleviated the stress, decreased my luggage weight and increased my love of travel.

The three-colour method

When preparing for a trip, we want to pack an appropriate wardrobe that will suit all possible scenarios but we don't always know what the weather and local environment will be like and what the holiday will entail from day to day. We often prioritise comfort – after all, travelling can be a time to relax and unwind, and may involve a lot of walking – but you might also want something a bit dressier for a dinner or show you're attending.

However, we also don't want to overpack. There's nothing worse than lugging around an overstuffed suitcase that you can barely lift off the baggage carousel. How often have you come home from a holiday only to have worn half of what you packed? We ideally want to pack only what we need, which is a cohesive mix-and-match wardrobe. It sounds simple but can be elusive in reality! As such, I rely on a couple of packing methods.

Gretchelle Quiambao popularised the 'Rule of Three' for packing as far back as 2014. While she suggests packing three of each core item (shoes, pants, tops, et cetera), the three-colour method limits your colour palette, and it is something I've been using for a while. It is pretty self-explanatory: choose just three key colours to pack – and though it might sound a bit dull (it's not – see below!), this method really changed how I feel about packing for any kind of holiday.

Using this method means packing less but, ironically, it gives you more options. The first benefit I discovered was that having fewer choices reduces confusion. It helps me pack with greater ease and efficiency because it rules out anything in my wardrobe that isn't these three colours. It also brings immediate clarity to how the pieces all work together.

For example, when I first employed the three-colour method, I chose black, beige and white. These are colours I own a lot of, so I was able to choose pieces from different categories of my wardrobe. I suggest you start with a combination of classic colours in your wardrobe too, which for you might be navy, grey and white, or blue denim, black and tan, or grey, black and white.

I do apply some flexibility to the three-colour method with accessories (shoes, belts, jewellery, bags, etc.) and allow a couple of wardrobe staples such as a classic white t-shirt, a striped Breton top or an extra pair of jeans. Adding these not only allows you to inject your unique style personality into your travel wardrobe but also provides even more options to mix and match, while still maintaining the ease and functionality of a limited colour palette.

So, in addition to my travel capsule of black, beige and white, I threw in a red and white Breton stripe long-sleeve knit, a pair of red sandals and a leopard-print crossbody bag, all of which added personality and interest to my base items.

All up, I packed just 14 items:

1. beige blazer
2. black blazer
3. black dress
4. black jeans
5. black sandals
6. black shorts
7. white jeans
8. white t-shirt
9. red and white Breton stripe knit
10. red sandals
11. white ballet flats
12. black bag
13. black belt
14. leopard-print bag.

This allowed me so many outfit options, some of which were:

Outfit 1: black shorts, white t-shirt, white ballet flats, black belt, beige blazer, black bag.

Outfit 2: black shorts, red and white Breton stripe, white ballet flats, leopard-print bag.

Outfit 3: black jeans, black blazer, white t-shirt, red sandals, leopard-print bag.

Outfit 4: black dress, beige blazer, black sandals, leopard-print bag.

Outfit 5: white jeans, black belt, white t-shirt, beige blazer, red sandals, black bag.

Refreshing your palette

Limiting your packing wardrobe to three colours doesn't mean compromising on your love of colour. When travelling with a colourful capsule, you can use more neutral accessories in white, black or denim. For example, after having great success with my first few attempts at the three-colour method using classic colour combinations, I graduated to using other colours from my wardrobe. I've since used olive green, baby blue and cinnamon as my three primary colours, adding white accessories to tie everything together and a pop of colour via a bold yellow knit to add visual interest and variety. This is how my packing looks when using those these three as my colour set.

Three-colour: olive green, baby blue and cinnamon

- blue jeans
- blue shirt
- cinnamon blazer
- cinnamon pants
- olive dress
- olive long vest
- olive shorts
- white bag
- white ballet flats
- white sandals
- white tank
- yellow knit

Some of my outfits for this collection included:

Outfit 1: light blue shirt, cinnamon pants and blazer, white sandals, yellow knit over shoulders.

Outfit 2: blue jeans, white tank, olive long vest, white ballet flats, white bag.

Outfit 3: olive dress, cinnamon blazer, yellow knit around waist, white sandals, white bag.

Outfit 4: olive dress, cinnamon blazer, white bag, white sandals.

Outfit 5: olive shorts, blue shirt, olive green vest, white ballet flats, white bag.

Outfit 6: blue jeans, blue shirt, yellow knit over shoulders, white ballet flats.

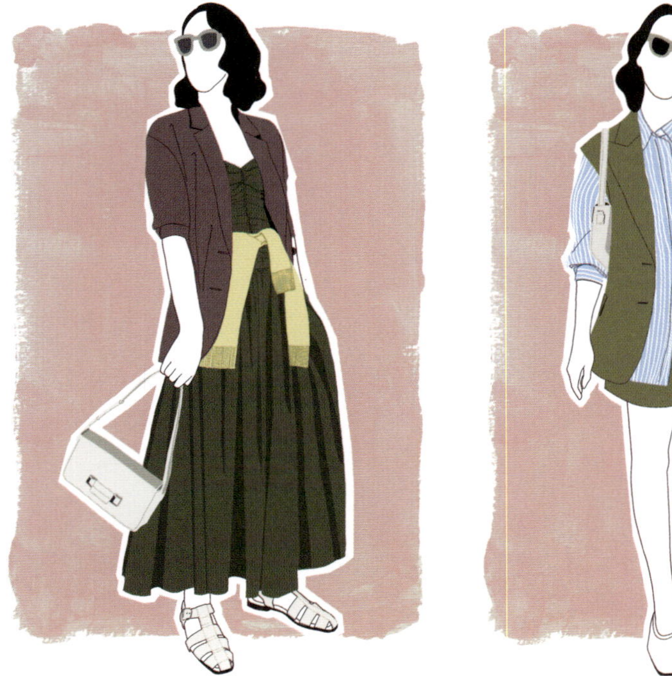

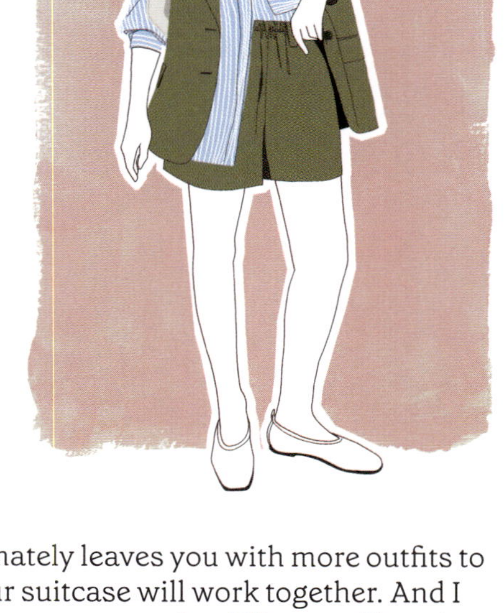

The three-colour packing method ultimately leaves you with more outfits to choose from because everything in your suitcase will work together. And I guarantee you won't end up looking the same every day. What you'll see is a versatile, stylish wardrobe that takes up less physical and mental space and gives you more time to enjoy whatever you're packing for.

I've used the three-colour method to pack for many trips from a long weekend to a week-long holiday, and I'm quite confident I could use it to pack for longer trips too. Try it first for a short holiday and see how you go.

The 5-4-3-2-1 packing method

This is another packing method I first came across via social media (like many good style hacks) and while it's difficult to pinpoint exactly who invented it, one of the first to popularise it was blogger Geneva Vanderzeil. As with all things style, it has evolved over the years as it provides lots of variations and flexibility to personalise it. There are many interpretations of the method but, essentially, the 5-4-3-2-1 refers to the number of items you take in any one category. The categories and allocated numbers are up to you but they're usually determined by the type of holiday you're going on, as I'll show you.

The advantage of this method, much like the three-colour method, is that it sets some boundaries for your packing, encouraging you to be more considered and intentional with your selections. It's actually quite fun and I have discovered that, because of these parameters, I am more likely to select things from my wardrobe that I really like because I'm 'forced' to be somewhat ruthless. The 5-4-3-2-1 method allows me to pack strategically, while easing the burden of overpacking.

Packing for New Zealand

The first time I tried it was for a seven-day holiday in New Zealand. This was a good test because the trip required clothing for cold temperatures, meaning coats/jackets, knitwear, pants and covered-in shoes. Layering was the goal, and the 5-4-3-2-1 method allowed for just that. For this trip I interpreted the 'one' category as being able to take one item of a few things.

How my New Zealand wardrobe looked for seven days:

5 × knitwear: cream turtleneck, lilac knit, red turtleneck, rust knit, green knit.

4 × shirts: magenta shirt, denim shirt, blue and white stripe shirt, blue and rust stripe shirt.

3 × pants: blue jeans, burgundy striped trackpants, green striped trackpants.

2 × blazers: brown check blazer, houndstooth blazer.

3 pairs of shoes: taupe sneakers, white ballet flats, red sneakers.

1 × coat, 1 × t-shirt, 1 × scarf, 1 × handbag: green coat, blue and brown check scarf, brown bag, white tee.

This gave me several outfits including:

Outfit 1: green striped trackpants, brown check blazer, cream turtleneck, rust knit over shoulders, taupe sneakers, brown bag.

↙ **Outfit 2:** burgundy striped trackpants, white ballet flats, magenta shirt over white tee, houndstooth blazer, lilac knit over shoulders, brown bag.

Outfit 3: brown check blazer, blue jeans, red sneakers, red turtleneck, blue and brown scarf, brown bag.

Outfit 4: burgundy striped trackpants, taupe sneakers, cream turtleneck, houndstooth blazer, green knit over shoulders, blue and white shirt, brown bag.

↘ **Outfit 5:** green coat, taupe sneakers, blue jeans, blue and rust shirt, rust knit over shoulders, brown bag.

Outfit 6: green striped trackpants, white ballet flats, denim shirt worn unbuttoned over white t-shirt, brown check blazer, green knit over shoulders, brown bag.

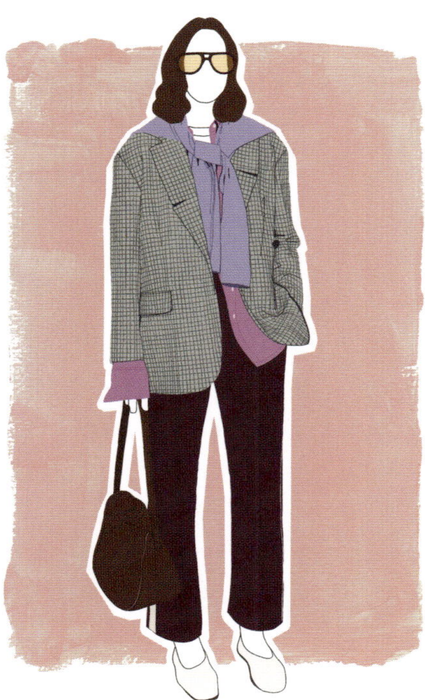

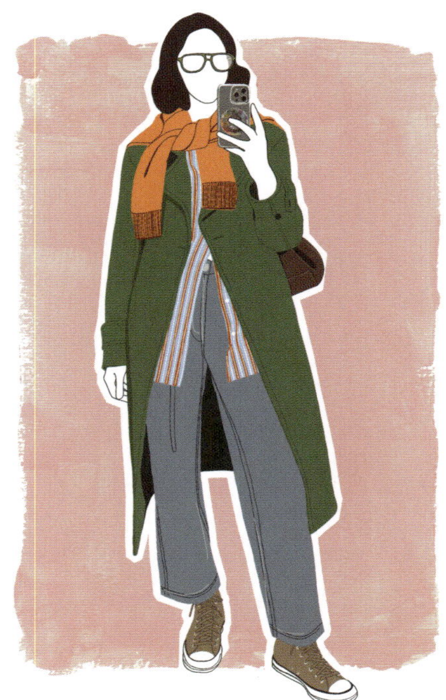

There are no restrictions on colour for this method but on this trip I decided
not to pack any black. And guess what? Because I had a formula to guide me,
I was easily able to select things from my wardrobe that worked together,
even though I packed a variety of different colours. The method allows for
countless outfit combinations – probably more than you really need for a
week-long trip – but without needing an abundance of clothes.

Packing for other trips

Let's apply this method to a couple of other holiday types and climates.

How my summer in Thailand wardrobe looked for ten days:

- 5 × dresses
- 4 × sleeveless tops
- 3 × shorts
- 2 × bathers
- 1 × hat, 1 × linen shirt, 1 × sarong, 1 × tote
- Other: 2 pairs of sandals.

How my spring in Japan wardrobe looked for seven days:

- 5 × t-shirts
- 4 × jeans/skirts
- 3 × jackets
- 2 × sneakers
- 1 × knit, 1 × handbag, 1 × dress.

Remember, these methods are guidelines to help minimise the angst around
travel packing, not rules! No one is going to arrest you at customs if you
don't adhere to them precisely. They are simply designed to help reduce
the overwhelm when it comes to vacation packing, and they've definitely
worked for me.

Time to pack!

I have a few recommendations to assist you with packing like a pro, no matter what method you use. I recommend you clear your bed and place a white sheet on top. Now you've got the perfect canvas to start planning your travel capsule. Alternatively, if you have access to a portable clothes rack, use that instead. They really are a great tool to help you plan your outfits (not just for travel but every day!).

If you've completed the activities earlier in the book, you'll have collected a healthy number of images that inspire your personal style or are outfits that you've worn yourself and felt your best in. I want you to refer to these when packing for your next holiday, because they have already helped you to determine your style personality.

You can also use your phone to take photos of outfit combinations before your trip. If you've got the time (and energy), taking photos will not only be useful in the planning process but also while you're away because all the hard work and thinking has already been done. You can simply look back through the photos and pick an outfit for the day!

First, place all your selections on your bed or rack. You don't have to be too deliberate about this at first, just use them as 'placeholders' to get the process started. It's amazing how quickly you'll start to see your wardrobe coming together, or not!

Once your bed or rack is full of the pieces you initially think will work, start to visualise how pieces are going to work together, assembling your outfits one by one. As you do this, you'll start to identify which pieces are the 'outliers', i.e. pieces that only work with one outfit, such as a top that only goes with one pair of trousers or a pair of shoes that only goes with one skirt, and you can confidently omit them from the packing equation, choosing something that is more versatile instead.

Sometimes a simple flat-lay on my bed provides enough visual representation to satisfy my styling needs, and other times I like to try on the outfits to assess in the mirror. Do whatever works for you depending on your time constraints or energy levels. And remember, whatever packing method works best for you, always focus on choosing items that you feel like yourself in.

17. WEAR YOUR WARDROBE

This might sound like a silly title for a chapter – after all what else are we supposed to do with our wardrobes, eat them?! But in fact, many of us do not wear our wardrobes nearly enough.

I have visited thousands of wardrobes, and sometimes even stood in front of my own, brimming with clothing but lacking the inspiration to put it all together. Wardrobes full of beautiful pieces, some with the tags still attached, some still in their shopping bag and others gathering dust in the back of the closet; clothes that don't fit or are 'too good' to wear, clothes that were bought while travelling overseas or on sale, or hand-me-downs. And don't get me started on the clothes that would be perfect if only you lived in a different climate, had a different job, a different lifestyle . . . a different life!

In this final chapter, with your style tools in hand, we bring together all the ideas, concepts and inspiration in *STYLED* to use the clothes in your wardrobe for the sole purpose you bought them for in the first place – to wear them! It's time to wear your clothes, and I'm going to show you how. Let's troubleshoot some of the common reasons we don't wear our clothes so you can start getting the most out of your wardrobe!

Clothes that are 'too dressy' or 'too nice'

Have you got something in your wardrobe that you love but feel it's 'too dressy' or 'too nice' to wear most days of your life? I've always been of the belief that I'd rather be overdressed than underdressed, whether it's to go to work, to a sporting event, on holiday or even to the supermarket. Now, this doesn't mean I wear a ballgown to the grocery store but I might wear a beautiful coat to the football instead of my puffer jacket, paired with jeans and sneakers. Who cares if you're 'only' picking the kids up from school? Wear a blazer with your jeans instead of a daggy jumper. So what if you're 'only' hanging out at a friend's house? You can still wear a nice dress. Who cares if you're 'only' popping out to the shops? Tailored pants will look great with your sneakers and t-shirt. The more you wear these 'dressy' pieces, the more comfortable you'll feel reaching for them any day of the week.

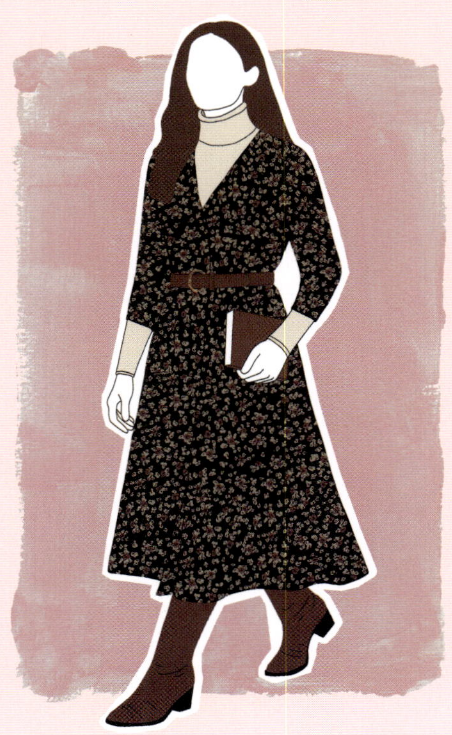

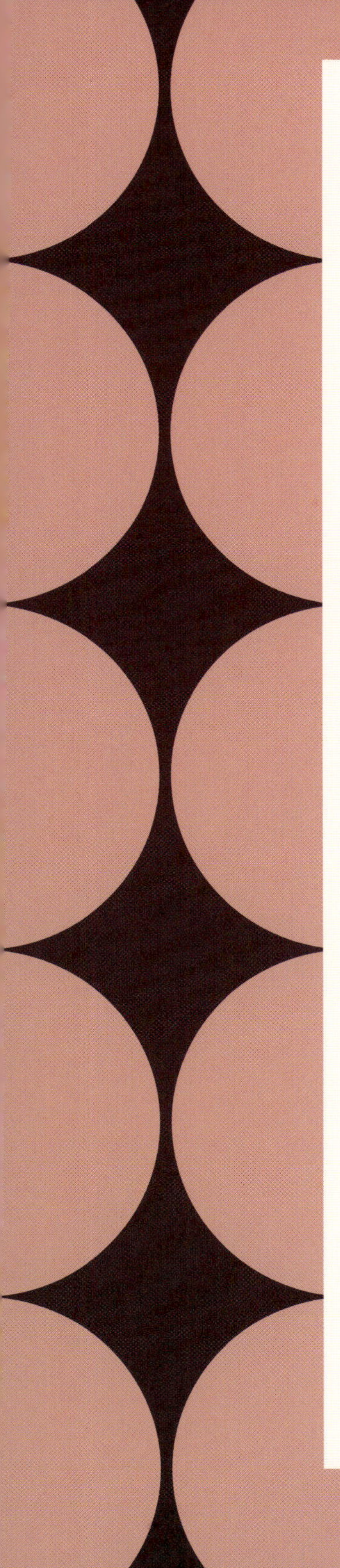

Activity: Rethink, restyle, re-wear

What you need:

pen and paper

clothes from your wardrobe

Let's get straight into it with a practical activity to rethink those pieces you love but don't wear enough. Perhaps the way you used to style them doesn't work for your current lifestyle, so they sit gathering dust. Perhaps they're the pieces you usually only wear on summer holidays, leaving them unworn for eleven months of the year. Or perhaps the style feels outdated and no longer aligns with your personal style. Well, it's time to have a rethink.

Take one item from your wardrobe that you love and want to wear more regularly:

1. Identify its 'regular' purpose (i.e. a work pant).

2. Identify a new purpose for it (i.e. a casual pant).

3. Write down at least one new way to style the item to serve its new purpose.

4. Wear that outfit ASAP!

Example 1

Tailored navy pants typically worn for work, styled with a patterned blouse, cream heels and a navy blazer. These pants could be styled with:

- sneakers, an oversized jumper and a casual tote bag

- flats, a graphic tee, a trench coat and a bum bag

- an off-the-shoulder top, strappy heels, a blazer over the shoulders and a clutch.

Example 2

Floral A-line brocade midi-skirt typically worn out for dinner, styled with a fitted top tucked in, with Mary-Janes and stockings. This skirt could be styled with:

- a t-shirt and sandals

- knee-high boots and an oversized rollneck jumper, untucked

- sneakers, a tank and a denim jacket.

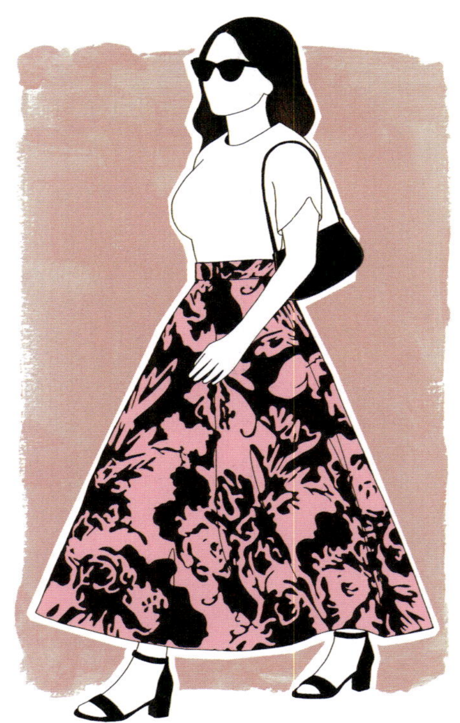

Example 3

Silk summer dress with shoestring straps typically worn in summer with sandals. This dress could be styled:

- under a cropped knit with ankle boots

- over a turtleneck, under a longline vest, with a waist belt, patterned tights and boots

- over a white t-shirt with combat boots and a denim jacket.

Can you see how many possibilities there are already in your wardrobe? With just a little imagination and creativity, you can find new ways to wear these 'too nice' pieces every day. Just give it a try. It might not end up being a combination you have the confidence to wear out of the house but, by experimenting, you will start to open your mind to more possibilities. Don't forget to take photos of the outfits you create. Whether you wear them or not, they'll be a great reminder of the endless wardrobe potential you have at your disposal.

Clothes that no longer feel like 'you'

It came to me one day that certain items in my wardrobe no longer felt like 'me' anymore. They were pieces that I still loved but wasn't wearing, pieces that, when I put them on, I'd take them off again. I had come to the conclusion that they no longer aligned with my style but that was until I thought about how to *repurpose* them.

Over my years as a stylist, I've taught many clients how to declassify their wardrobes (see Chapter 4), showing them how to style items in various ways for maximum versatility and functionality. This approach helps ensure both a highly workable wardrobe as well as a cost-effective one. But the art of repurposing one's clothes to prolong their lifespan is a little different and, in my experience, rather liberating!

I'll use my collection of Zimmermann dresses as an example. I wore these dresses a lot over an almost ten-year period. I loved them and they felt very 'me' at a certain period of my career. They made a statement and were effortless, feminine and the ultimate 'one and done' item in my wardrobe, needing only some fab shoes, a bag and some jewellery or a belt for me to feel amazing. But over the years, as my style evolved, they became less and less a part of my everyday style. I reached for them rarely, and when I did, I'd usually take them off again. They didn't feel right. I still loved them but they no longer aligned with my style personality or my wardrobe purpose. I found myself wondering if I'd ever wear them again. When I did some thinking, the answer became a surprising yes: I repurposed them.

Instead of trying time and again (and failing) to style these dresses for my everyday life in Melbourne, I instead styled them to suit a new purpose in my life – summer vacations – and I instantly felt more 'me' in them.

↗ Zimmermann paisley midi-dress

Original purpose: work

New purpose: holiday

The dresses, not only styled in a more casual way with flat sandals, the belt removed and a casual handbag but also for a more casual purpose, now felt aligned to how I wanted to feel on holidays. Still polished and modern but relaxed.

The bonus of the repurpose strategy is that I have a new addition to my holiday wardrobe without having to buy something new. Here are a few more examples of items I've repurposed from clients' wardrobes.

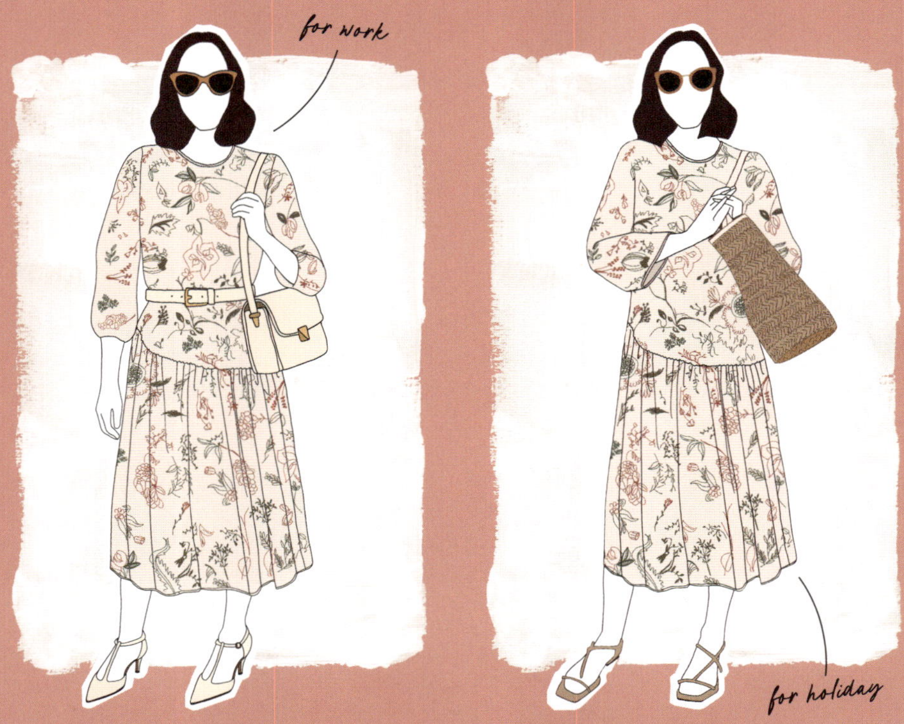

Classic camel knee-length trench coat

Original purpose: worn as an overcoat to the office over a pants suit with stilettos and a briefcase for work.

New purpose: worn as an overcoat on the weekend with blue jeans, a hoodie, sneakers and a crossbody bag.

Valentino Rockstud heels

Original purpose: worn for a night on the town with a black, fitted knee-length dress and a fringed black clutch.

New purpose: worn to a mid-week dinner with friends with boyfriend jeans, a white tank, a chunky gold necklace and a fringed black clutch.

Black leather biker jacket

Original purpose: watching live music, worn with black skinny jeans, black ankle boots, a band tee and a black bum bag.

New purpose: for casual Friday at work, worn with black, tailored wide-leg pants, black loafers, a black turtleneck and a black handbag.

Clothes that are dated or no longer fit

There are many reasons why it's difficult to let go of certain pieces from our wardrobes. We may have paid a lot for them or perhaps they were inherited from a loved one. Maybe they evoke fond memories, or we used to feel fabulous wearing them! But now, perhaps a hemline is too short, a sleeve too tight or a button too shiny, and the style feels a bit dated.

Another way to get value from what you already own is to consider remodelling something – altering a garment to give it a new lease on life. If you still love the fabric or something about an old favourite, consider whether you can adjust it somehow to make it feel more like you today.

Michele

Michele's wardrobe was an eclectic assortment of high street and high-end pieces she'd bought second-hand or had inherited from family members. She showed me some old favourite dresses that she still loved but was no longer wearing. She couldn't quite put her finger on why, as she loved the colours, patterns and fabric.

When she tried them on for me, I identified what the problems were. The dresses, which Michele used to wear with tights and knee-high boots, were no longer suited to her current preference for high-rise, wide-leg jeans and trousers. The dresses were also a lot shorter than what she preferred to wear today.

'Why don't we turn them into tops?' I suggested. 'That way you can wear them tucked in to your jeans and trousers.'

'I never thought of that! I love that idea!' she replied.

Michele took a few of these dresses to her local tailor to get them shortened and hemmed. She sent me a photo after she collected them. She was wearing one of her dresses with the most amazing collar and pattern, neatly tucked in to her favourite pair of high-rise corduroy jeans.

A simple remodel, an elaborate new life and, most importantly, Michele was wearing her clothes!

Rehome your clothes

What happens when you do all the right things – rethink, repurpose, remodel – but something just doesn't feel right anymore? When do you know it's time to let something go from your wardrobe?

I've been helping clients edit their wardrobes for many years, and one of the hardest things for people to do is to let go of clothing they once loved. But it's okay to find a new home for these things and to pass them on to someone else to enjoy, just like you did. We have more avenues than ever for selling or donating our pre-loved clothing. The second-hand market is growing at an exponential rate with demand for pre-loved fashion booming. Online resell platforms, consignment stores, clothes swaps, charity donations, op shops, markets . . . there are endless options when it comes to giving your unwanted clothing a new home. When considering if it's time to let go of something you no longer wear, ask yourself:

- Why haven't I worn it?

- How did I feel the last time I wore it?

- How do I feel about it today?

- Would I wear it today and feel like myself? Why/why not?

When I work with clients, I listen carefully to the language they use about their clothes. It's very revealing! When you stop to ask yourself these questions, it will become very clear how something makes you feel, and why it might be time to let it go. Remember, there's always interim options, such as a box under your bed or the wardrobe in the spare room, where you can store things that you're not quite ready or willing to part with. These items might be things that just don't fit now, crush items that are no longer 'on trend' but you still love them, or pieces you spent a lot of money on and parting with them just makes you feel sick. That's okay.

However, if you reach for an item of clothing and the first three words you use to describe how you feel about it have negative connotations, then your answer is clear . . . it's time to say goodbye!

Anne

Anne's small wardrobe was full-to-bursting with clothes she barely wore. She was a classic example of someone wearing 20 per cent of her wardrobe 80 per cent of the time. Her high-rotation pieces were a modern pair of wide-leg jeans (her current faves), some cashmere knitwear and ballet flats. She didn't need a lot of clothes because she wore a uniform at work and led a casual life, preferring to catch up with friends for brunch and lunch rather than fancy restaurants for dinner but she wanted to wear what she had more often.

I asked Anne to show me something that she hadn't worn for ages. She grabbed a pair of faded blue jeans with a drop crotch and textured fade lines (what's known in fashion circles as 'whiskering') across the hips. 'So, tell me about these,' I said.

'I bought these back when I was studying, and I used to think I looked so cool in them. I wore them with a leather jacket and studded ankle boots (Chloé dupes) but I haven't worn them since I started working and that was nearly ten years ago!'

'How do you feel about them now?' I asked. 'Do you still think they're cool?'

She shook her head. 'I want to like them but every time I put them on, they don't feel like me anymore; they feel too sloppy, too relaxed. I don't like how the drop crotch gives me a "saggy bum" look. I prefer my new jeans that sit high on my waist and give me more shape. These feel very dated.'

Anne did not mention one positive thing about the jeans. She associated only negative thoughts and feelings about the jeans. They were not something that could be rethought, repurposed or remodelled, so out they went. She just needed my 'permission' to let them go.

Rani

Rani had just celebrated her fortieth birthday and a job promotion and wanted to elevate her professional wardrobe. She had worked in the corporate world since her early twenties but hadn't really updated her work look since then. It was time to step it up.

'Show me a typical outfit you'd wear to work today,' I said.

Rani pulled out some old suits she'd been wearing since she first started working over fifteen years ago. The suits were very characteristic of the time they were purchased: short, fitted blazers, low-rise straight-leg trousers and above-the-knee pencil skirts. She liked to team these with more feminine blouses made of soft fabrics and usually a bright colour or pattern.

'How do you feel in these suits today?' I asked.

'I still feel like the junior lawyer who turned up to her first day of work. Even though I remember feeling so confident in them at the time, I don't feel like they reflect who I am today, nor the progress I've made in my profession and the senior position I've worked so hard to get. When I see my colleagues in more modern corporate wear I feel a bit dowdy and dated, even though I'm a lot younger than many of them.'

Describing these pieces to me was enough information for Rani to see that it was time for these suits to go. Like Anne's old jeans, there was no way to update the suits to be more aligned with the Rani of today and because she associated only negative thoughts and feelings about her corporate image, it was time to create a new one.

Say goodbye to clothes that have had their day

The significant thing to note in these examples is that these clothes *were* worn – a lot! Anne wore her drop-crotch jeans almost every day at university and Rani wore her suits for fifteen years. It's important to remember this if you're feeling guilty about moving something on from your wardrobe. Think to yourself: did I love it when I wore it? Did I wear it a lot? Did it serve my wardrobe purpose at the time? If the answers are yes, then don't feel guilty for parting with these items. They served you well and now it's time for someone else to enjoy them.

Repeat the exercise in this chapter as often as you like, with as many items as you can that you are not wearing regularly. If you can't rethink something by pairing it with different items to better suit your current wardrobe purpose and style personality, see if you can repurpose or remodel it. If not, say goodbye and welcome the newfound space in your wardrobe – and your life!

Welcome the
newfound space
in your wardrobe –
and your life!

Our clothes are
the armour we wear
to *face the day*,
be it good or bad.

STYLED YOUR WAY

With *STYLED* I hope that I have instilled in you the tools, knowledge and conviction to use and wear clothes to present the person you want to be. It's easy to brush off personal style as superficial, frivolous and insignificant in the scheme of life but I'll bring you back to one of the first points I made. We all must get dressed, every day. Our clothes are the armour we wear to face the day, be it good or bad. On days when we're not feeling our best, when things are hard and life feels overwhelming, one of the things we have control over is our clothes and how they make us feel.

Your life will evolve, and with that, your wardrobe will too. Each of you reading this book today has already experienced significant change throughout your life, and there is likely more to come. You might change jobs, move countries, change partners, perhaps have a baby, or lose or gain weight, and your tastes will change too as you get older. It's a good thing to want to change, learn and grow, in all aspects of life, and your personal style is no different.

I wrote *STYLED* to help you navigate these changes and learn to trust your instincts, always – regardless of what's 'in' or 'out', or your age, size, height, shape or budget. I hope that I've challenged you to take risks, to dress to please no one but yourself, that I've encouraged you to wear more of your wardrobe, to shop less and to buy things that truly align with who you are and what you want your clothes to say about you.

I hope that by identifying your style personality, determining your wardrobe purpose, organising and declassifying your wardrobe, letting go of 'the rules', embracing your shape and learning how to shop for the life you lead today, you're feeling more empowered than ever to build outfits that make you feel great, every day.

If I were to ask you now, 'Closet full of clothes and nothing to wear?', I hope you would respond emphatically with a 'Hell no!' because you're on your way to building a wardrobe of clothes with *everything* to wear. Now, go forth and get dressed, feel great and be *STYLED*.

PENGUIN BOOKS

UK | USA | Canada | Ireland | Australia
India | New Zealand | South Africa | China

Penguin Books is part of the Penguin Random House group of companies
whose addresses can be found at global.penguinrandomhouse.com

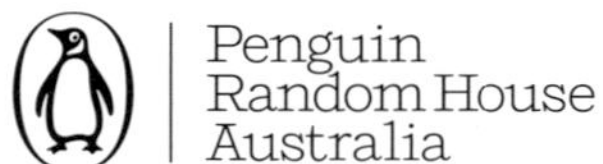

Penguin
Random House
Australia

First published by Penguin Books in 2025

Copyright © Sally Mackinnon 2025
Illustrations copyright © Juliet Sulejmani 2025

The moral right of the author has been asserted.

Cover and internal design by Andy Warren © Penguin Random House Australia Pty Ltd
Typeset in Faktum and Grenette Pro by Post Pre-press, Australia

Printed and bound by 1010 Printing International Ltd, China

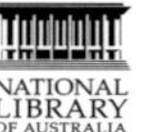

A catalogue record for this
book is available from the
National Library of Australia

ISBN 978 1 76134 920 1

We at Penguin Random House Australia acknowledge that Aboriginal and Torres Strait Islander
peoples are the Traditional Custodians and the first storytellers of the lands on which we live
and work. We honour Aboriginal and Torres Strait Islander peoples' continuous connection to
Country, waters, skies and communities. We celebrate Aboriginal and Torres Strait Islander
stories, traditions and living cultures, and we pay our respects to Elders past and present.

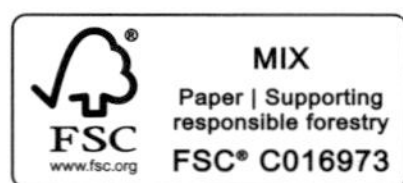